BEYOND FOODS

The Handbook of Functional Nutrition

BARBARA SWANSON

BALBOA PRESS
A DIVISION OF HAY HOUSE

Copyright © 2016 Barbara Kay Swanson.
Graphic Illustrations with Julie Winsberg

All rights reserved. No part of this book may be used or reproduced by any means, graphic, electronic, or mechanical, including photocopying, recording, taping or by any information storage retrieval system without the written permission of the author except in the case of brief quotations embodied in critical articles and reviews.

Balboa Press books may be ordered through booksellers or by contacting:

Balboa Press
A Division of Hay House
1663 Liberty Drive
Bloomington, IN 47403
www.balboapress.com
1 (877) 407-4847

Because of the dynamic nature of the Internet, any web addresses or links contained in this book may have changed since publication and may no longer be valid. The views expressed in this work are solely those of the author and do not necessarily reflect the views of the publisher, and the publisher hereby disclaims any responsibility for them.

The author of this book does not dispense medical advice or prescribe the use of any technique as a form of treatment for physical, emotional, or medical problems without the advice of a physician, either directly or indirectly. The intent of the author is only to offer information of a general nature to help you in your quest for emotional and spiritual well-being. In the event you use any of the information in this book for yourself, which is your constitutional right, the author and the publisher assume no responsibility for your actions.

Any people depicted in stock imagery provided by Thinkstock are models, and such images are being used for illustrative purposes only.
Certain stock imagery © Thinkstock.

Print information available on the last page.

ISBN: 978-1-5043-5482-0 (sc)
ISBN: 978-1-5043-5484-4 (hc)
ISBN: 978-1-5043-5483-7 (e)

Library of Congress Control Number: 2016905618

Balboa Press rev. date: 04/27/2016

CONTENTS

Preface 7
Acknowledgments 11

Section 1: What Happened to Our Food?

Chapter 1 The History of Food 13
              Naturalwashing and Greenwashing 18
              Functional Nutrition 21

Chapter 2 Food Choices Today 23
              Why Won't Junk Foods Nourish Me? 23
              Isolates Versus Wholefoods 24
              Nanotech Nutrients 25
              Medicine Versus Natural Healing 28

Chapter 3 Three Secrets of a Healthy Diet 30

Section 2: The Four Building Blocks of Functional Nutrition

Chapter 4 Your Complex Body Made Simple 40
              Beyond Foods 40
              The Four Building Blocks of Functional Nutrition 42

Chapter 5 Building Block 1—Superfoods 45
              The Raw Materials of Cellular Health 45
              Why Superfoods? 46
              Essential Nutrients: Vitamins 47
              Essential Nutrients: Minerals 49
              Essential Nutrients: Amino Acids 53
              Essential Nutrients: Essential Fatty Acids ... 57
              Essential Nutrients: Important Phytonutrients 59

Summary	63
What You Can Do	64

Chapter 6 Building Block 2: Digestive Nutrients 69
- Enzymes 71
- Digestive Nutrients: Probiotics 79
- Summary 87
- What You Can Do 88

Chapter 7 Building Block 3: Antioxidants to Protect Cellular Function 90
- ROS Free Radicals 91
- Oxidative Stress 94
- Antioxidants 95
- Nutrient Antioxidants 97
- The Immune Connection 98
- Summary 100
- What You Can Do 101

Chapter 8 Building Block 4: Regenerative Nutrients 103
- Epigenetics 104
- Telomeres 106
- Adult Stem Cells 109
- Summary 111
- What You Can Do 112

Conclusion 115
Bibliography 120

The doctor of the future will give no medication, but will interest his patients in the care of the human frame, diet and in the cause and prevention of disease.

—Thomas A. Edison

Prevention is better than cure.

—Desiderius Erasmus

PREFACE

> Just imagine, how much easier our lives would be if we were born with a "user guide or owner's manual" which could tell us what to eat and how to live healthy.
>
> —Erika M. Szabo

This book is just that—an easy-to-understand handbook of what your diet must contain for a healthy body. You won't need a degree to understand this information, nor will you be asked to completely change your life and diet (although I am sure there are shifts you may wish to make after reading this). *Knowledge is power!*

Over the last twenty-two years of working as a health consultant, my focus has always been to help people achieve a greater level of physical, mental, and emotional well-being through lifestyle choices, with an emphasis on the benefits of whole, ancient foods and food-based supplements. I see, nearly on a daily basis, the struggle people have trying to make the best, most affordable, and simplest choices for their health needs.

I am fortunate to have been taught by a wide variety of mentors and icons in the alternative health and nutrition field. This wide-lens view kept me from thinking there is only one right way to eat for health.

I have had the privilege of learning directly from Viktoras Kulvinskas, cofounder of the Hippocrates Health Institute, author of the health classic *Survival in the 21st Century*, and father of the living foods movement. I have worked closely with several teachers from the renowned Kushi Institute, home of the modern macrobiotic movement.

I routinely consult with people with widely varying dietary choices, including vegans and vegetarians, athletes and trainers who expound the paleo diet and even people who eat fast food weekly and want to figure out better choices.

Through the process of doing hundreds of personal consultations, I have seen the great need people have for a basic nutritional education to help them understand how to determine if a diet change or supplement would be beneficial—or not.

Over the space of a fifteen-year (and counting) research journey, I have read books about nutritional science and studied different nutritional and lifestyle alternatives to Western medicine. I gathered information from other researchers on specific health topics, such as digestive health, enzymatic nutrition, and how specific nutrients affect various organs and systems. I learned how light is turned into the food we eat and about *food energetics*. I also reviewed hundreds of human clinical trials, epidemiological studies, *in vivo* and *in vitro** studies, and many double-blind peer-reviewed scientific studies.

After thousands of hours of research, I came to realize that there is an underlying order to how foods and supplements work to create better health. This knowledge helps explain the powerful benefits of using whole, wild foods as an essential component of a healthy diet.

Why Diets Don't Work

The usual thread in "going on a diet" is that each tries to offer a single, simple solution to a specific problem—e.g., how to lose weight, have more energy, cleanse toxins, or create more muscle mass. Each need

---

* *In vivo* refers to a scientific test done on a living animal. *In vitro* refers to tests done outside a living body (culture dish, test tube, etc).

is approached as a separate issue. People are taught to find *the* diet or *the* supplement that will work for what they want *at that moment*.

The truth is unless your diet fulfills the ongoing basic nutrient requirements of all your cells and organ systems, you will likely fail at meeting any long-term dietary goal.

A diet is not a fad you use for a few weeks or months. It is how you provide the nutrients and micronutrients that support your body's physical needs right now—and next year, and in ten years. In fact, no matter what physical state you are in at the moment, no matter what your specific health situation, the nutritional factors you need for life must be in the foods and supplements you eat.

This book doesn't offer or recommend a specific diet, other than one that is filled with real, whole foods and whole food supplements, adding in wild and ancient foods as much as possible.

This book is the distilled result of knowledge gleaned from dozens of indigenous diets, backed by hundreds of scientific studies from widely varying sources. It presents you with a simple and complete system that helps you understand how to eat for the *four building blocks of functional nutrition*.

Beyond Foods offers a new way to look at both diet and supplementation. You won't read how to eat to lose weight, lower inflammation, or get rid of belly fat *as if they are separate problems*.

Realize this—you don't need a supplement to lose weight, another supplement to lower inflammation, and yet a different program to detox and cleanse. You need to eat a diet and use powerful whole-food-based supplements filled with the whole-food nutrients that support cellular health and body systems. Your body will then do the rest of the work to retain (or regain) good health to the best of your genetic capacity. And science has shown that even your own genetic code can be rewritten, to some degree, via a healthy diet and lifestyle choices.

My goal is to make sure that you know what your body needs on the cellular level—regardless of the type of diet you choose. I want to help you choose supplements that are not a waste of money or worse, actually cause a nutritional imbalance.

Once you understand what you need in your diet—and why—you can make informed choices that will give you the benefits you need.

You will learn what to eat in order to allow the innate intelligence of your genetics to work to their fullest potential ...

You will learn how to eat *beyond foods*.

Barbara Swanson

ACKNOWLEDGMENTS

I have more people to thank than it is possible to list. However, I wish to publicly acknowledge those without whom this book would not exist.

First and foremost, I wish to thank Donia Al'Alawi. This book would not exist without her input, including ideas and years of collaboration, inspiration, and insight on the resolution of how to, as best as possible, communicate in a simple way some of the very complex ideas involved in the workings of functional nutrition.

I also wish to thank the entire field of business peers with whom I work. There are hundreds of you, and while I don't have room to list your names, you are all important.

Of special note are my friends and much more—you know who you are. I wish to thank my mentor in understanding the deep history of foods, Steve Gagne; the father of living foods and my dear friend, Viktoras Kulvinskas; Katharine Clark, a living avatar of the live foods movement; and fellow author (and one who is far more accomplished than I) Dr. Jeffrey Bruno, whose research on earth's most ancient food will enlighten our world.

And most of all, I would like to express deep love and gratitude for my children, who have supported me no matter what path I have walked.

Disclaimer

All statements in this book are those of the author and based on her research and beliefs. The statements in this book have not been reviewed by the FDA. This book is not intended to prevent, diagnose, treat, or cure any disease or disease process. See your qualified medical professional if you have concerns regarding your health.

SECTION 1

What Happened to Our Food?

It should be simple: make a grocery list, buy the food, make a meal—and be nourished. Not so long ago, that was true. Today, however, we really do live in a different world, and our eating choices have to be more conscious if we are to actually be *nourished* by what we eat.

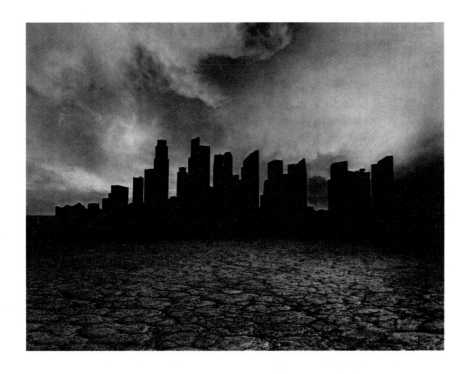

Chapter 1
The History of Food

For more than five thousand years, humans have used foods to prevent or ease the symptoms of various diseases. The old adage "An apple a day keeps the doctor away" has recently been scientifically validated.

The truth is that modern medicine has a history of pooh-poohing old wives' tales, only to then discover they are based on verifiable scientific facts. This attitude is ironic, considering that using foods as the first choice to heal or prevent diseases was laid out by the father of modern medicine, Hippocrates, more than two thousand years ago.

In the modern world, it is important to find a great whole-foods micronutrient-support program. Sadly, most people today eat a diet filled with foods that not only do not but *cannot* actually nourish them.

Even seventy-five years ago, you didn't really need to think about what you ate—or even know what foods nourished your body or how. If you ate it, you would be nourished.

Until the mid-twentieth century, the majority of foods eaten on a daily basis were homegrown or locally sourced. Seventy-five years ago, the foods we ate were raised without an overload of herbicides or pesticides. There were no concerns with GMO contamination.

Milk wasn't homogenized for shelf life and then pasteurized to protect us from the results of cattle being raised in unhealthy conditions. Cattle weren't fed antibiotics, hormones, and steroids to increase productivity. Until the 1950s, practices such as shipping from massive farming complexes and using chemical fertilizers, herbicides, and pesticides were not the norm.

Beyond Foods

After World War II, we experienced a dramatic downward shift in nourishment from our daily foods: the proliferation of convenience foods, fast foods, and foods shipped from around the world, rather than foods sourced locally.

Our diets moved away from freshly harvested, freshly prepared whole foods into convenient and fast foods. Today the average fast-food meal has about eighty synthetic additives to enhance flavor and texture. Any single *one* of these additives could cause slight changes in brain chemistry. Added up together, they can spell disaster for healthy brain function, especially in young, still-developing brains—yet doctors wonder about the increase in autistic and hyperactive behavior and say they can find no cause.

We now eat far more processed foods and synthetics than have been determined to be safe. I—and many health educators and health professionals—believe the side effects we deal with due to the addition of these additives and chemicals include dramatic increases in chronic diseases and a lowering of our standard of health at younger and younger ages. We see upward climbs in profound brain dysfunction and other diseases at early ages. ADD/ADHD, ASD (autistic spectrum disorder), juvenile diabetes, and asthma are just the tip of the visible health dysfunctions increasing in our children.

It's not only foods we have to worry about. There are increasing numbers of lab-created "nutrients" and synthetic supplements. They seem to offer everything you need. But synthetic nutrients, isolated amino acids, processed fatty acids, minerals from rock, or any type of genetically modified (GMO) foods don't—*can't*—offer wholesome nutrition.

The reason for this is simple: *we don't assimilate them.* Our bodies cannot easily utilize isolated nutrients, and some the body won't assimilate at all, let alone recognize as food.

In the last decade, people have woken up to the problem of not being able to find actual, real, healthy nutrition in the foods they eat. This has spurred a huge increase in sales of natural, green, and organic foods and supplements. Sales of supplements and organic foods are in the billions—and both categories have been growing yearly for over a decade. *This isn't a trend—it is a movement.* As such, manufacturers want in on the sales action, even if what they offer isn't really all that healthy.

There are trends within this movement toward healthier foods and supplements. Often these trends are a reaction to the problems caused by eating too much processed and fast food. For example, a scientific study will show a problem with salt or fat, but rather than saying, "Don't eat processed and fast foods, loaded with salt and trans fats", the advice is to remove that single nutrient, which is also found in healthy forms in whole foods. What all these trends have in common is this: if people will pay for something, a manufacturer will create it then sell and promote it.

Often this leads to some manufacturer making a "safer, better" food—usually through replacing the nutritional culprit with a different processed ingredient, which often winds up being far worse for your health. Let's look at a few examples.

One of the first trends was to limit salt. Indeed, high levels of regular table salt are deadly! However, rather than providing education on the need for drinking healthy amounts of good water, Americans were advised to simply eat low-sodium diets. Sodium continues to be a concern for many, primarily because most processed foods and restaurant-chain meals contain obscene amounts of salt as a cheap flavor enhancer for low-quality ingredients. Salt substitutes came into being, but information and understanding about the need for healthy salt is not readily available and information on the dangers of salt substitutes is hard to find.

Fast Fix: If you use boxed or canned foods or go to fast-food restaurants weekly, begin by replacing a single meal a week with whole foods, such as vegetables, fruits, whole grains, beans and rice that you purchase and cook yourself. Use flavoring spices to replace salt. Spices like paprika and mustard work with nearly any meal. Add garlic and other aromatics to add flavor. You will be in control of the amount of salt you add. Use a natural, unheated salt, such as Celtic Gray, and discover just how little salt you really need to add great flavor.

Next came the trend to limit fats. And like the no-salt/low-salt fad, people are still looking for a low-fat/no-fat number on their food—and too often pay next to no attention to any other information on the label, such as synthetic additives needed for flavor. Manufacturers have created chemicals that will prevent fat absorption—which are now found to lead to vitamin deficiencies and other severe digestive problems. Only this year has the government stepped in to actually limit sales of trans fats—processed fats that are known to lead to chronic inflammation, which is a root of hundreds of diseases and conditions. In recent years, the need for healthy fats has spurred people to add "good" fats back in through the practice of adding omega fatty acid supplements.

Fast Fix: Eat real foods with good fats in moderate amounts. Half of a raw avocado or a small handful of seeds and nuts are fantastic sources of healthy fats; either will provide an amazing energy boost in the afternoon. At only sixty-six calories, two teaspoons of virgin olive oil or virgin coconut butter adds a ton of flavor to a salad, cooked vegetables, popcorn, or even granola.

Refined sugar—and its real dangers—has been a problem for decades. But in recent advertising campaigns, the differences between highly processed sugars and sugars that naturally occur in fruit and other minimally processed sugar sources (such as honey) are minimized and even outright denied. Instead of limiting or eliminating soda and candy, people use *deadly* synthetic substitutes, which are finally being proven to be not only dangerous but ineffective at helping control weight loss.

Fast Fix: Use one or two teaspoons of raw honey, real maple syrup, or yacon syrup to flavor foods. Eat fresh, raw fruits. Eat a snack with fiber if you want something sweet; fiber slows the absorption of sugar into your bloodstream. If you crave juice, make it raw and fresh; the cost will keep you from drinking more than is good for you. In addition, the fiber is healthy.

We are now in the midst of a trend to remove gluten from all foods. Many people believe they have celiac disease, a very severe immune response to a protein found in gluten, which is always in wheat and often in other grains. However, there is a fundamental and large difference between true celiac disease and gluten sensitivity. I personally believe the dramatic increase in gluten reactions is a by-product of the fact that nearly all nonorganic grains contain deadly pesticide residue, leading to chronic inflammation. And some grains are now also genetically modified (GMO). GMO grains have protein sequences that can stimulate immune reactions similar to those associated with celiac disease. But the issue of a GMO-protein intolerance or inflammation caused by pesticides or other toxins mimicking gluten sensitivity is barely acknowledged. As a result, people are paying double and triple the normal cost of an item for that gluten-free product they think they need.

Fast Fix: Use all organic grains to minimize exposure to pesticide residue and GMOs, and see if this helps with your grain-sensitivity reactions. Instead of buying processed grain foods (e.g., pasta, breads, and so on), choose whole grains, such as steel-cut oats, quinoa, and brown rice. Eat no more than 1 cup of any grain per day. Eat sprouted grains when available. Note—if you have true celiac disease, you need to be 100 percent gluten free.

Naturalwashing and Greenwashing

Greenwashing is the term used to describe the practice by which a manufacturer uses meaningless terms and words coupled with impressive marketing to give the impression their product is environmentally safe and friendly, natural, and good for you—even if their product is known to be toxic. Examples of this are Coca-Cola using plant-based plastic in their new bottles and Clorox purchasing Burt's Bees to sweeten their corporate profile.

Naturalwashing is the supplement equivalent of greenwashing. Words like *natural* and *plant-derived* sound encouraging, but they *have no actual meaning* with regards to the safety or quality of the product. Examples of naturalwashing include:

- *Natural*—This word has no legal meaning when it comes to supplements or personal care. Basically, if it is on our planet, we can claim it is "natural." For example, Crystal Light, which is mostly synthetic flavors and aspartame, is called natural.
- *Plant-derived*—This can mean just about anything, since plants form the majority of edible products in one way or another. For example, petrochemicals are plant-derived.

- *Contains no artificial (flavorings, ingredients, and so on)*: Since the word *natural* has no legal definition, the definition of *artificial* is nearly as meaningless.
- _____ *blend* (proprietary protein blend, trademarked vegetable blend, and so on)—Trademarked or proprietary, blends are a great way to hide the fact that the main ingredient within that blend might be cheap filler. It works like this. US labeling laws require that ingredients are listed in order, from greatest amount to least—with the exception of proprietary blends. All ingredients within a trademarked or proprietary blend are allowed to be listed in any order the manufacturer desires. For example, a powdered vegetable drink has only one organic superfood, and it represents the least amount in the formula. On a regular label, it would have to be the last ingredient on the label. However, if the manufacturer creates a proprietary blend, that lone organic superfood can now be listed first instead of last.
- *Contains 100 percent recommended daily allowance (RDA) of vitamins*—Increasingly, supplement manufacturers will add a few real food ingredients to mostly synthetic products in order to woo people who are looking for real food formulas. People see foods like blueberry powder or kale and assume the list of synthetic vitamins that follows are from the foods listed. To my knowledge—and I have looked at hundreds of food-based vitamin formulas—no 100 percent food formula contains exactly 100 percent of all vitamins. If a drink blend is created from various dried foods, they will not contain exactly 100 percent of all vitamins. They might contain *more* than 100 percent of a very few vitamins (for example, a drink with camu camu may contain several hundred percent of vitamin C's RDA). When you see vitamins listed, followed by similarly high percentages of the RDA for them all, you can safely assume the

product is fortified with synthetic versions of those vitamins. For example, legally, you can create a 100 percent synthetic vitamin formula, add it to a fermentation vat with a whole-food base, and call your product a 100 percent whole-food vitamin formula. There are at least three very popular whole-food vitamin formulas that do exactly this.

- *Clinically proven*—"Clinically proven" can mean something ... or nothing at all. Consumers are aware that marketing and product promotional materials are filled with deceitful statements. So they are cued in to look for some sort of scientific validation, and the gold standard is a scientific study or clinical trial. I want to clarify that I am *not* saying trials and studies are worthless—not at all. A peer-reviewed double-blind placebo-controlled study or good clinical trial can offer valuable insights into whether a product contains an ingredient (nutrient) that offers certain specific benefits. However, both trials and studies also have potential flaws with regards to determining the value of food-based supplements. They include the following.
    1. Most studies focus on a single nutrient, and it is often synthetic. This allows the cause and results of the study to be easier to track and verify. However, whole foods have multiple nutrients, working in concert. Therefore, the result of a study done on a single nutrient may not reflect the entire range of benefits found in a whole food.
    2. Many studies on specific formulas or products are done for a week or two, on a few people. This is a cheap way to get a clinical trial without an extreme cost.
    3. A clinical trial or scientific study is, by definition, a narrow snapshot of the whole. It can be extremely valuable to learn, for example, that a key nutrient is an anti-inflammatory. What is the outcome of this? Which

is actually better for you—a product that is highly processed to extract that single *proven* nutrient or the whole food containing that nutrient and *hundreds* of others which have not yet been studied?

4. Clinical studies and trials are extremely expensive. There is a lot of private money to back most decent scientific studies or trials. Ask yourself, "Who makes the money back?" The answer—drug companies. The dependence on this type of science as the only *good* science, with the dismissal of all other forms of proof as being irrelevant or *bad* science is directly correlated with the rise of drugs and drug use to replace foods as our primary way to handle health and prevent disease. Foods are not easily quantified or qualified via the narrow parameters that are inherent in a study.

- *Phony testimonials*—People love to hear success stories, and companies know this. You can go from product to product online, and you will see that many of the personal testimonials use *exactly* the same wording, with only the name (first name only) changed. These are not real. These are lures, designed to hook you into trying a product that may not even be safe for you to use, much less good for you.

Functional Nutrition

This book will help you navigate through the minefield we just looked at by teaching you the four simple tenets of functional nutrition. *Functional nutrition is the basic philosophy that the human body is designed with the ability to grow, regulate, repair, and defend itself when given natural, whole-food nutrition.*

Beyond Foods

Functional nutrition recognizes the scientific fact that in order for our body's cells, organs, and systems to function normally, we have certain basic biological or physiological *needs* that must be met via our diet. Functional nutrition states that if we provide the correct raw materials (nutrients) via the foods we eat (our diet), the human body will naturally function at its highest health potential.

As long as we meet these nutritional raw material needs effectively and consistently, the body thrives—known as good health and vitality.

The following chapters help you understand what nutrients foods must contain in order to actually nourish your body and how they do so, based on the principles of functional nutrition.

This book does not espouse any single type of diet as *the one*—raw, macrobiotic, vegan, vegetarian, or paleo. I don't believe that you must eradicate all the foods you enjoy—even if they are less than ideal nutritionally. This book is a simple guide, with simple explanations, to the foods and supplements that contain the nutrients you must have in order to meet your body's cellular needs; then the food choices are up to you.

This book is a layperson's resource. I have deliberately kept the principles and explanations as simple (yet accurate) as possible.

Information and details on any single one of the four building blocks could easily stand alone as a book of this size (and in fact, I will be writing more detailed guides to each of these building blocks). While there are hundreds of scientific studies, clinical trials, and resource books used in my research, *Beyond Foods* is created to function as a basic, easy-to-use handbook on how functional nutrition works to create good health, vital energy, and healthy aging.

Chapter 2
Food Choices Today

There are two major categories of foods we can choose to eat from to satisfy our hunger.

Real foods are as is from nature, in a whole and complete form. There are three qualities of real foods:

- *Wild-harvested foods* are the highest quality in terms of nutrient potential. They exist naturally in an uncultivated state and are wild-harvested in a variety of ways.
- *Organic foods* offer nutrients which are cultivated without contamination by GMOs, chemical fertilizers, pesticides, or other toxins.
- *Agribusiness foods* are those foods cultivated with chemical fertilizers plus pesticides, herbicides, and fungicides. Animals are raised using steroids, hormones, and antibiotics. GMOs are increasingly common. Eating foods with these additives and processes can be dangerous to your health.

Junk foods include all foods that have been highly processed, synthesized, denatured, isolated, fragmented, or refined or processed using high heat, chemicals, or solvents. This definition probably includes foods you may consider healthy, such as light olive oil, as well as most isolated nutrient supplements.

Why Won't Junk Foods Nourish Me?

When you are hungry for a cheeseburger or a piece of pie instead of a stir-fry or carrot, it is your mind telling you what tastes good. Your body has a completely different way to determine what it wants—i.e., *needs*—in order to create good health.

Beyond Foods

Your body asks you for a diet that will generate energy to support growth (calories such as you find in carbohydrate-rich foods like whole grains—or pies); for amino acids to support muscle strength (such as you would find in protein-rich foods like beans or nuts—or a burger); for essential fatty acids to nourish your brain and nerves (such as you would find in seeds, nuts, or avocados—or cheese pizza); or for other micronutrients, such as vitamins or minerals (as you find in carrots or a stir-fry). Your body, if you listen, will crave foods that offer a wide range of potent nutritional components that protect the body's cells and tissues and support essential metabolic functions.

Think about it this way. When a cheeseburger, pie, or a carrot is thoroughly digested and absorbed into the bloodstream, is it still the cheeseburger, pie, or carrot? *Of course not.* It has now been broken down into one or more distinct groups of nutrients and nutritional cofactors.

To function in an optimal health state, you must daily supply your body with nearly fifty essential nutrients. These essential nutrients cannot be produced by your body; they must be supplied by foods. These essential nutrients include at least twenty-two minerals, thirteen vitamins, ten essential amino acids, and two essential fatty acids.

Getting your micronutrient needs met through whole-food nutrition is essential.

Isolates Versus Wholefoods

In fact, several studies suggest that isolated supplements are not as *assimilable* (usable by your body) as nutrients found in whole foods. (You will learn more about the importance of assimilation in the next chapter.)

One example is a study using synthetic vitamin E (alpha tocopherol). It showed that the isolated form of the vitamin is not as assimilable as natural E complexes. And that is no surprise, as our bodies actually use pro-vitamin A (beta-carotenes, a pigment found in carrots, algae, and other fruits and vegetables) and with good probiotic bacteria and other cofactors found in food, make vitamin E in our digestive tract. There are other studies that even suggest that supplementation via the use of vitamin isolates can actually lead to symptoms of vitamin deficiencies.

There is no doubt that when you eat a whole food, you gain nutritionally. The reason for this—the reason you need whole foods and whole-food-based supplements—is that *every single nutrient acts in concert with a host of cofactors*. Amino acids need other amino acids and minerals; minerals need amino acids and essential fatty acids; and vitamins need minerals. Add to this the need for your body to have a host of probiotic bacteria and their intrinsic factors in order to assimilate the nutrients found in your foods, and you begin to see why any lab-created, synthetic, or isolated nutrient program is bound to come up short.

Nanotech Nutrients

Another development in food science is nanotech nutrition. A nanoparticle (NP) is extremely small. Nanotechnology works on a molecular level to change the structure of a nutrient. *In fact, a nutrient requires very intense and high-level processing to create the molecular and structural changes that are necessary to make a nano-sized particle.*

Some foods and their nutrients are naturally nano-sized, such as nutrients in single-celled foods like microalgae. However, any nanotech-based lab-created formula will contain NP nutrients, which have been significantly changed on the molecular level in order to make them into something not found in nature.

One example of this type of very intense processing is when oil-soluble ingredients are changed by nanotechnology so that they are able to be absorbed in water. In my opinion, there is real danger in using what is essentially a new way to uptake nutrients at a cellular level. Taking supplements that are not properly formulated (balanced, with safe restraints placed on their bioavailability) is like force-feeding. Yet we are still trying to figure out exactly how different micronutrients and minerals interact and act on our cells—even our DNA—with normal-sized whole-food nutrients.

In fact, there is grave concern about the safety of untested nanotech nutritionals, and studies indicate evidence of ongoing toxicity due to our body being unable to recognize and safely eliminate NP nutrients via normal biological channels.

Even universally recognized, highly useful minerals, like calcium or iron, are toxic if the dosage is too high. For this reason, I personally avoid any NP nutrient products.

Food as Medicine

Modern civilization has moved far away from the knowledge that food is medicine. This is not a surprise; according to a National Institutes of Health (NIH) study published in 2008, only 30 percent of the medical schools in the United States even require a separate nutrition course at all—and some schools consider it an elective! On average, a doctor receives less than twenty-five hours of nutritional education in twelve years of study of how the human body functions. *This is horrifying when you really pause to consider that without food, absolutely not a*

single cell of your body will have the necessary raw materials for life, much less a healthy life.

Today, most people are taught—and believe—they have to fix pain, sadness, disorders, and diseases with drugs. Consider these statistics.

- Nearly half of all Americans take at least one drug a month.
- Nearly thirty percent of all Americans take more than one drug.
- Twenty percent of American children are on a prescription drug.
- The number-one prescription for US adolescents is for central nervous system stimulants—drugs that directly and often permanently affect brain function.

It is ironic that statistically, the better health care you have (the more regularly you see a doctor), the *more* prescriptions you use. What this means is that *having a doctor doesn't actually improve your health*; it simply makes it more likely you are on a drug for the symptoms of being unhealthy.

Yet despite the increase in drug use for diseases—the vast majority of which deal with symptoms only, not causes—people don't feel better, and they know it. Twice as many people rate their health as "less than ideal" than did ten years ago. And Americans are not only unhealthy, they are unhappy. The number-one type of prescription for those between the ages of twenty-five to forty-five are antidepressants.

The real truth? People don't see food as an optional way to increase health and well-being. For most, eating is just a problem to solve. Food is viewed as something to avoid or indulge in, not as a tool that will enhance life quality.

Beyond Foods

Medicine Versus Natural Healing

Let's compare taking a drug to the process of how the body uses nutrients to heal. If you have a headache, a doctor might recommend an anti-inflammatory pain reliever, such as aspirin. The headache disappears, and everyone is happy. The symptom (a headache) was treated, and often, no further thought is given to the episode.

With natural healing, you ask questions. *What caused the headache?* The treatment is then focused on removing the imbalance, nutrient deficiency, lifestyle situation, or toxicity that actually caused the problem.

Based on the treatment prescribed, if we applied the natural healing model to the Western medicine treatment and resultant headache *cure*, we would conclude the headache was caused by an aspirin deficiency. We know that isn't the cause!

Deficiency of any of the nearly fifty essentials nutrients that we need in our diets can result in slow but certain physical deterioration. Most of the foods grown on commercial farms today are produced by chemical fertilization in depleted soil. The result is food that looks pretty but does not always supply the nutrients our bodies need for good health.

In addition, hundreds of chemicals have been added to our food to color it, change its taste, keep its shape, help it resist mold, and assist it to have a longer shelf life in the grocery store—i.e., make it look attractive, not keep it nutritious. Except for foods that are certified organic, whole, and "as is", these chemicals are in nearly any food we purchase. This guarantees we will have ongoing toxicity complicating our health.

In this book, we introduce the *Four Building Blocks of Functional Nutrition*. These offer a way to show you how to look beyond symptoms and actually use nutrition to help redress the cause of a problem, not just cover up any symptoms. Our health model helps you know how to access the functional foods that support your body's natural health. By knowing the meaning of functional nutrition and knowing what building block nutrients are essential for ongoing good health, you are empowered to make the best choices for your needs today, tomorrow, and in your future.

Chapter 3
Three Secrets of a Healthy Diet

Secret #1: Anything is better than nothing.

A lot of diets are severely restrictive, either of calories or of food types. A lot of supplement protocols require you to use several different supplements, adding new ones for each problem. Many times, you are told you won't get any benefits if you don't follow the exact diet or protocol.

We certainly recommend restricting some foods (notably sugar, fast foods, and processed foods) and definitely recommend certain supplements. However, over twenty-five years and hundreds of consultations, we have seen that the main reason people quit is either they simply can't continue to follow the restrictions or they can't afford the regimen of supplements.

And when you don't understand why to choose this supplement versus that one, the choice is either follow directions or quit altogether.

While this book helps explain to you the nutrients you must have to live a healthier life—even if your other habits are not yet ideal—the truth is that you do *not* have to change everything in order to start seeing benefits.

The bottom line is *making any positive change is better than attempting no change!*

Testimonial #1: Stephanie's† Story

I remember working with Stephanie. She had been tentatively diagnosed with multiple sclerosis (MS) six months previously, after twelve months of increasingly poor health.

She smoked, drank diet soda incessantly, had an extremely high stress job, and often ate fast or prepackaged foods because she had no energy to prepare meals.

She came to me after having tried several different supplements and was willing to do anything except stop smoking or change her job. She understood that fast and prepackaged convenience foods weren't healthy but simply didn't have the energy or time to try to cook from scratch.

Rather than make her wrong or refuse to work with her, we did what we could. The first change was to remove all the diet drinks and foods that contained aspartame or any other synthetic sweetener. I got her to commit to drinking at least two quarts of spring water daily to replace the soda. She then began to use whole, wild-food-based supplements. She agreed to eat a salad daily, even if it was from a buffet at a fast-food chain.

She felt even worse for nearly three weeks, with the worst symptoms being headaches and aching muscles. She blamed the new supplements, and I assured her that it was likely a cleansing reaction to removing aspartame.

She began to feel better at about four weeks, and as the weeks went on, she began to feel *a lot* better—she had more energy, no headaches,

---

† All names have been changed to protect the privacy of our clients.

less anger and sadness, and no muscle weakness. On a return visit to her doctor after three months, testing showed no clinical signs of MS.

Now, we will never know if this was a coincidence. However, Stephanie felt fantastic, after eighteen months of feeling increasingly weak, exhausted, and depressed.

As a bonus no one expected, she quit smoking! She told me that despite herself, she simply couldn't stand the way cigarettes made her feel anymore.

Once she quit smoking, her health took a huge leap forward. She lost about fifteen pounds that she had put on over a ten-year period. She was healthier and happier than she could remember being in years.

This story illustrates the second secret.

Secret # 2: No symptom or problem exists in a vacuum; all parts of your life are connected and interconnected.

This is a truth most of us realize, at least unconsciously. The stress of our job is offset when we go to the gym or for a run. A long night out leads to fuzzed thinking and slow reflexes. An angry confrontation feels less overwhelming when we hold our cat or hug a child.

Whatever is going on in your life—positive or negative, emotional or physical—can and will affect other areas in your life.

Often, the less healthy, unconscious ways we try to handle ongoing stress or problems are culprits that sabotage our good health. These include the following.

- binging on sugar or chips when we are bored, hungry, tired, or overwhelmed
- deciding that with no energy or time to make a meal, a fast-food dinner won't hurt us
- eating a bar for breakfast because we overslept, then buying a soda for lunch because there wasn't time to make food for work and no money in our budget to buy it at a restaurant; crashing at 2:00 p.m. and consuming a candy bar and energy drink then crashing again on the way home from work and stopping to get a protein fix with a double bacon cheeseburger, then deciding to also get an order of fries and a milk shake because, after all, we hadn't really eaten all day...

The reality is any one of these situations might occur occasionally with no real lasting health impact. But people get into habits, and habits create our health, for better or worse.

There is a proven, scientific connection between digestion and brain function. There is a connection between brain function and emotion.

There is a connection between nutrients and brain chemistry.

There is a connection between brain chemistry and our ability to cope with stress.

Ultimately, the very way you are able to think, feel, process, and make choices can be dramatically affected by a nutritional lack of which you may not even be aware.

And it is the second precept, *no problem exists in a vacuum*, that makes the first precept, *any positive change is better than none*, work.

Beyond Foods

Testimonial #2: Ivy's Issue

An example is Ivy's story. Ivy is a longtime acquaintance. We were not close friends but certainly friendly, as we are both artists in our small community.

Several years ago, I noticed her car at a stop sign as I was crossing the street.

I hadn't seen her in several months, and I was stunned. Ivy had always been vibrant, a lovely woman with striking features made all the lovelier because of the energy she exuded as effortlessly as breathing. She was an artist, owned a thriving real estate company, and was on several civic committees. Now she appeared shrunken in upon herself with dull skin, dull hair, and dull eyes.

I was so shocked that I walked up to her car and motioned for her to lower her window. I asked her what was wrong, and she looked at me as if I were a stranger. Without asking, I went around, got in the other front seat, and told her to go park somewhere we could talk. She told me she didn't have time in a flat voice, as if she didn't really care, and then parked anyway.

When I asked her what was wrong, she told me she had been fighting a severe case of chronic fatigue syndrome (CFS). Since the last time I had seen her, maybe six months previously, she had gained about twenty pounds and, worse, she had lost her light—that indefinable sense of vitality that made her beautiful to everyone.

She explained that she could barely function; her company was in trouble because she couldn't work. She slept sixteen to twenty hours a day and still felt exhausted. The doctors had no relief for her, and nothing she had tried resulted in any benefits (not that she stuck with anything for long—it was too much effort).

I asked if this illness just came out of the blue or if she had been feeling poorly for some time and hadn't told anyone. Her explanation is the perfect example of *precept 2—no symptom or problem occurs in a vacuum*.

She told me her husband of many decades, the love of her life—her soul mate—had died about eight months previously, after a long fight with cancer. She had been his sole caregiver, and he had died in her arms. She said she had felt emptied out emotionally but was at peace with his passing.

Then, about two months after his death, while she was changing their bedroom around, a heavy table fell on her big toe.

She said that immediately, beyond the pain of a broken toe, she felt her energy collapse as if she were a balloon with a pinprick. She went to bed and had mostly been there ever since, unable to summon the energy to move forward.

So with Ivy, we have someone who had been dealing with severe emotional stress for several months and then suffered a shocking injury. The injury itself wasn't severe, but the shock was. She had no reserves left to combat the pain, and it sent her entire being spiraling downward. The connection between emotional exhaustion, physical pain, and immune function played out in terrible symmetry.

Using whole wild foods, we bolstered her body reserves. The benefits and results surprised even us. Within a month, she was back at work. Within two months, she was working six to eight hours a day and sleeping eight to nine hours a night, and the lights were back on in her eyes. She regained her joy of life and the spark that makes her unique.

Ivy's story illustrates the power of our body to heal, given the right raw materials. This power is literally a miracle, which I never take for granted.

Secret #3: The raw materials for health and regeneration are found in whole foods and whole-food supplements.

Our physical bodies are built from essential nutrients found in *foods*. For many thousands of years, our bodies have created and refined incredibly complex, interrelated biological systems that are dependent upon the raw materials foods provide. I believe that when food has been split apart, fragmented, and processed, the body goes looking for the missing parts. For example, if you eat fragmented wheat, like white bread, where the bran and germ of the whole grain have been removed, your body will still be hungry and seek the missing part of the food (e.g., something with fiber or crunch). Unfortunately, that crunch is often found in yet another processed food, like chips.

Many—if not most—vitamin formulas are completely synthesized versions—created in a lab.

Why?

Cost. It is much more expensive to handle real foods to create a vitamin formula. It is much costlier to keep them from degrading.

Many—if not most—mineral formulas are created from powdered rocks.

Why?

Cost. It is much cheaper to grind and clean rock than to produce plant-based mineral supplements.

Many—if not most—supplements contain one or both of the above, in addition to fractionated or isolated food nutrients.

Why?

Cost. It is simply easier to manufacture in a chemical lab than go through the quality control required to use whole, live foods.

And *you* pay the price for this with supplements that do not work as nature intended.

Testimonial #3: Laurel's Energy

Laurel had always eaten well. She lived rurally, which helped minimize stress, and had a very active lifestyle. She had always been an outdoor sports person—hiking, jogging, camping, bicycling, cross-country skiing, boating, and more. As an artist and mother, she was creatively fulfilled.

The year Laurel turned forty-four, she completely ran out of energy. In her words: "I used to run daily; now I didn't even feel like going for a walk. I had 'brain fog.' In the mornings when I woke up, it seemed I was trying to look through a thin veil. I felt so weak some days that I should not have been driving. I was afraid that something was really wrong with me."

At a friend's suggestion, Laurel decided to see if adding wild foods and superfood supplements would make a difference in her energy levels.

Beyond Foods

She began by adding a wild algae superfood to her already clean diet. Within days, she noticed improvements in focus. She felt full after a meal and broke the snacking habit she had gotten into. Her hair stopped falling out.

And most important to her, some energy started to come back. She lost the brain fog that kept her from fully engaging in her life.

After several months of eating wild superfoods daily, she began to run five miles on her mountain trails every day. Today, at over sixty, she continues to have vibrant health and energy for her busy life as an artist and grandmother.

For Laurel, the additional powerful nutrients found in whole, wild foods was the nutritional boost her body needed to move forward into the next phase of healthy aging.

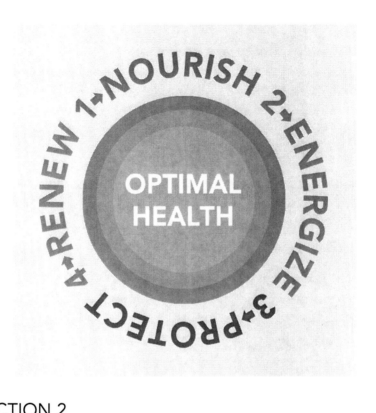

SECTION 2

The Four Building Blocks of Functional Nutrition

The *Four Building Blocks of Functional Nutrition* health model helps you understand the basic nutrient needs everybody has. This health model is based on millennia of humans using foods to support good health, the work of twentieth-century health pioneers who held tight to this knowledge, and scientific advances that help us explain why and how foods create health.

Chapter 4
Your Complex Body Made Simple

Your body is an amazing symphony of miraculous biological functions. From your uninterrupted heartbeat to breathing, from blinking to thinking, hundreds of thousands of biochemical actions occur every second without conscious awareness.

These nearly incomprehensibly complex interrelationships take years of intensive study to even partly understand. However, the truth of how your body uses nutrition can be rendered down to relatively simple roots.

The Four Building Blocks of Functional Nutrition are a layperson's breakdown of the supremely complex into simple concepts. It offers a simple yet accurate way to understand the roots of how nutrition works in your body.

Beyond Foods

Scientific studies demonstrate that foods and dietary choices have a tremendous effect on our health. More and more studies are proving the links between specific foods and positive benefits on numerous health-related conditions.

One example is a study done by Dr. Paresh Dadona, a diabetes specialist in Buffalo, New York, who measured the body's response to a typical fast-food breakfast.

"Levels of a C-reactive protein, an indicator of systemic inflammation, shot up 'within literally minutes.' … 'I was shocked,' he recalls, 'that a simple M*******'s meal that seems harmless enough—the sort of high-fat, high-carbohydrate meal that 1 in 4 Americans eats regularly—would have such a dramatic effect. And it lasted for hours."

Along with studies showing the detrimental effect of processed and sugary foods, science is proving the importance of certain key micronutrients. In fact, even our genetic expression is affected by nutrients—or the lack of them. Every single function of your body, from breathing to thinking to movement, is utterly dependent on raw materials from your diet. If you are not giving your body the essential raw materials, it cannot perform those functions.

Imagine you want to build a new house. What do you need?

First, you need money to pay for materials and labor. Next you need the raw materials to create the home—framing materials, insulation, roofing, electrical lines, plumbing lines, heating and cooling, flooring, and finish materials. Then you need an architect who can design a structure that can last. Lastly, you need skilled workers to build a sturdy structure.

Now, imagine that this house is your body. We are born with the architect and workers ready to go, every moment of every day, thanks to our genetic code. We have built-in blueprints for plumbing and electrical systems, as well as built-in heating, cooling, and ventilation. Some of us are born with better blueprints than others—this is where genetics plays its key role.

Where many of us have system failures, *and this begins in the womb*, is in providing the raw materials that will allow our architect and builders to create the most magnificent home possible. We fail at providing the "cash"—the healthy energy—to sustain our home once it is built.

Beyond Foods

Unfortunately, many people give their body the equivalent of sand, paper, and strings instead of providing brick, mortar, and nails. If you want to stay vibrantly healthy and age gracefully, the first thing you have to do is provide the raw materials your body requires.

The four building blocks model will help you answer these key questions:

- Do you eat foods that provide the building blocks of your electrical system (nerves and brain)?
- Do you have the nutrients essential for a clean plumbing system that doesn't back up (constipation), spring a leak (e.g., acid reflux or leaky-gut syndrome), or break down (indigestion and bowel problems)?
- Are you providing the raw materials to keep your frame (muscles and bones) from tearing down over time?
- Do you have the right currency (cellular energy) to allow all these actions to occur thousands of times daily?

The Four Building Blocks of Functional Nutrition

The four building blocks of functional nutrition are the four foundational nutrient groups that build and support your body's cells and systems. Each building block offers essential, specific benefits.

Each building block ties into and supports the others. Together, they support the strong cellular foundation we experience as energy, vitality, and radiant health.

Building Block 1: Superfoods

Nourish

A superfood is a whole food which acts as powerhouse of concentrated nutrients, offering a lot of micronutrients for comparatively few calories.

Building Block 2: Digestive Nutrients

Energize

Digestive nutrients help your body to correctly break down foods into usable elements. This means that individual nutrients in foods are more effectively absorbed into your blood, where they become the fuel for all the cells in your body. Friendly bacteria and food enzymes help to efficiently and completely turn food into energy for life.

Building Block 3: Antioxidants

Protect

Antioxidants are molecules that are able to safely neutralize free radicals. This helps protect your cells from premature aging because of the wear and tear of metabolism, toxins, and daily life.

Building Block 4: Regenerative Nutrients

Renew

Regenerative nutrients are those foods scientifically proven to enhance and support chromosomal health, healthy genetic expression, telomere length, and adult stem cell production.

Beyond Foods

Nourish, Energize, Protect, Renew.

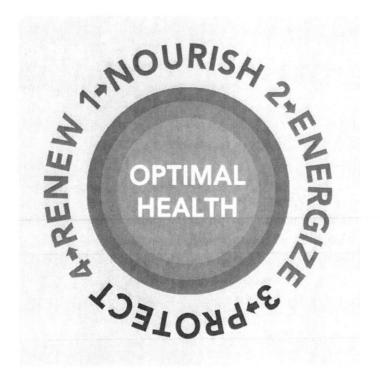

The Four Building Blocks of Functional Nutrition

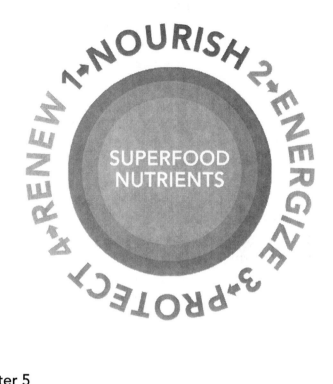

Chapter 5
Building Block 1—Superfoods

The Raw Materials of Cellular Health

Nutrition is often looked at only for your macronutrient needs—i.e., carbohydrates, fats, and proteins.

However, have you ever wondered why a fat is considered a good fat or a bad fat? Do you know the real difference between an energy-sustaining complex carbohydrate and a blood-sugar-spiking simple carbohydrate? Are you aware of how to choose the correct source of protein to fill your body's specific needs?

Beyond Foods

It is the micronutrient content of macronutrients that determines their value for your body. Healthy foods have macronutrients and sufficient micronutrients to provide for the underlying needs of our cells and body systems.

Many people are starving for micronutrients. Just because a food has calories from proteins, carbohydrates, or fats does *not* mean it will also have enough micronutrient nutrition for our body's cellular needs. For example:

- Over a dozen trace minerals are needed to support the endocrine system.
- Essential fatty acids are needed on a daily basis to feed and protect the fatty tissue of your brain and nervous system.
- Antioxidants are essential to help support healthy immune function and protect your cells from free radical damage.

Why Superfoods?

Superfood has become a buzzword to describe everything from watered-down sugary juices to lab-created synthetics. My definition of a superfood is as follows.

A superfood is an organically grown or wild-crafted whole food that offers a wide variety of micronutrients. Superfoods are powerhouses of concentrated nutrition, giving a lot of essential micronutrition for comparatively few calories.

Adding superfoods to your diet is extremely beneficial because of the lack of micronutrients in most Western diets. Corporate farming practices, processing, sterilization, and high heat along with other degrading additives have dramatically changed the micronutrient content of most foods. A great superfood will contain some or all of the following essential micronutrients.

- Minerals
- Vitamins and co-vitamins
- Essential Fatty Acids (EFAs)
- Essential Amino Acids
- Nucleotides
- Antioxidants, such as catechins or polyphenols
- Pigments like chlorophyll

All of these micronutrients are essential in order to grow, regenerate, and communicate on a cellular level. The body can compensate—for a while—for a lack in micronutrients. However, over time, these compensations have a domino effect on our health. Eventually it all comes tumbling down; symptom by symptom, your body will let you know it needs to be fed!

Essential Nutrients: Vitamins

Vitamins were first discovered in the early twentieth century by medical scientists who were searching for the root causes of certain diseases.

Today, sadly, medical science has focused outward for disease causes and cures, often recommending drugs as first choices rather than last chances.

Vitamins must be found within our diet. If they could be synthesized within our body, they wouldn't be called *vitamins*! In fact, one of the first discovered causes of disease was a vitamin deficiency. The following list is just a fraction of the vital functions vitamins perform.

- vitamins are essential for the correct formation of various life-sustaining enzymes.
- vitamins A and C are precursors to hormones that influence your genetic expression.
- B-complex vitamins are essential for healthy nerve function.
- B_{12} is essential for healthy genetic coding in your chromosomes.
- vitamins A, C, and E are potent antioxidants that help protect the body from damage caused by free radicals generated during metabolism or by exposure to toxins.

What about a "One a Day"?

Most multivitamins are cheaply made and almost always contain lab-synthesized vitamins. Vitamins manufactured in the laboratory, using isolated, synthetic, nonfood-based ingredients, are without the trace substances and cofactors that enable them to perform to their highest potential.

It is important to understand the concept of assimilation. *Assimilation* is the body's ability to actually recognize, uptake, and then utilize a nutrient. It is, in a way, a type of biological magic. Something outside of you becomes *who you are*. Our bodies have been fine-tuning how to access nutrients to support health and life for millennia, and they are very good at doing well with extremely minute amounts of key nutrients.

Multivitamins often contain many hundreds of times the recommended amount of a specific vitamin. If that form of vitamin will be poorly absorbed, as happens with synthetic vitamin isolates, then eating many times more than the needed amount *might* make sense.

However, the body often needs far less of the same vitamin when it is ingested via an easily assimilated whole foods that contains all the other nutrient cofactors necessary for that vitamin to function. An example of this synergy is in citrus fruits. They will have vitamin C *plus* rutin, bioflavonoids, and minerals—all of which are essential cofactors for absorption and utilization of this vitamin.

In general, when it comes to vitamins, less is better and food sources are *always* better assimilated than any type of isolate or synthetic vitamin. Our body is delicately balanced, a living collection of integrated systems with ongoing and subtle exchanges between the inside (our cells) and the outside (our food and environment). Too much of any one thing can be as bad for your health as too little. This means that taking more of one vitamin versus another can actually cause problems. Our body likes small amounts of easily absorbed and utilized micronutrients—as naturally occur in whole foods.

Essential Nutrients: Minerals

Minerals are necessary for the formation of dozens of chemicals in our body. They help regulate cellular metabolism. Minerals are critical components of enzymes and hormones, *and your body can't use any vitamin without the presence of minerals as cofactors*.

Micronutrient minerals are those needed in amounts of less than one hundred milligrams a day. There are seven minerals needed in larger amounts, including calcium, magnesium and phosphorus, but most minerals are considered micronutrients.

For an example of our body's underlying need for micro-minerals, let's consider its use of calcium.

We all know we need calcium. However, if you want to actually absorb and use calcium for healthy bones and joints, your body also needs:

Beyond Foods

- magnesium
- zinc
- copper

Plus you need:

- phosphorous to regulate calcium levels in the body
- sulfur and silica for the formation of collagen and elastin
- a cocktail of vitamins

And this is only in the context of bone and joint health!

Over twenty-two minerals have been proven necessary for human health. Yet many of the trace minerals we need could and would cause problems—and in some instances, even death—if taken in more than micro amounts.

The following are quotes from Senate Document 264, which was written in 1936, a time when food was generally fresher because more food was locally grown at that time and in general was less processed than it is today.

> ... It is bad news to learn from our leading authorities that 99 percent of the American people are deficient in these minerals, and that a marked deficiency in any one of the more important minerals actually results in DISEASE ... It is not commonly realized ... that ... Lacking vitamins, the system can make some use of minerals, but lacking minerals, vitamins are useless.

The need for minerals in order to have other nutrients function as your body needs is an example of the close interrelationships of all nutrients.

Chelated Versus Rock Minerals

If you take a regular multivitamin and mineral supplement, they likely contain isolated minerals—powdered rocks. These are natural minerals. To create a supplement, they are isolated, separated, cleaned, and purified.

The problem is that isolated rock minerals can actually lead to mineral imbalances in your body. The reason your body can't use the impressive list of minerals found in your supplements is because most often, rock-based minerals are inorganic—i.e., they have no carbon bonds. These carbon-based molecular bonds make the mineral "soft" or absorbable into your cells.

Inorganic minerals have molecules held together by very strong electric bonds. The scientific term for these strong, inorganic mineral kingdom bonds is *electrovalent*.

You can consume inorganic minerals, but your body has to do a lot of work to make them in any way assimilable. In order for minerals to actually be used by your body, they have to be connected to amino acids (which form organic molecules called peptides). This process is called *chelation*. Assimilability of inorganic minerals your body has to chelate will be very low, around 20 percent. Both colloidal and ionic minerals can be inorganic.

Often, your body will actually store inorganic minerals as toxins or try to eliminate them. Your body does not have the physical ability to easily convert inorganic hard minerals into usable organic soft minerals ... *but plants do.*

That's the beauty of plants as food. Plants process hard rock minerals through a biochemical process and turn them into chelated soft minerals. Aided by important soil-based bacteria, plants take minerals from the soil, break the electrovalent bonds, and then incorporate the minerals into their physical structure. Then, when we eat the plants (fruits, vegetables, seeds, and grains), our bodies are able to assimilate these chelated essential minerals.

Plants make the minerals soft or accessible for our bodies' cells.

Plants eat the mineral kingdom; we eat the plants.

Chelation allows minerals to pass through our cell membranes. The bonds formed by chelation are broken apart by your body as needed to be moved or converted into other physical structures.

Mineral uptake is a complex balancing act. Minerals do not work by themselves, only in relation to each other. This means that too much of any one mineral has the potential to throw off base entire mineral systems.

Let's take a closer look at how sensitive our bodies are in regard to mineral balances. Quoting from the book *Natural Healing with Foods* by Nancy Appleton:

> Let's look at two important minerals that work in direct relationship to one another: calcium and phosphorus. These minerals work best in the bloodstream in a relationship of 2.5-parts calcium to 1-part phosphorus ... This means that your ability to use the calcium in your system is phosphorus dependent: no matter how much calcium you have, you can only use it if there is enough phosphorus present to go with it.

Any additional calcium may become an excess that can cause a number of problems. Excess calcium may form hard deposits that irritate soft tissue; or sometimes excess calcium is stored in joints. Excess calcium in the arteries is unsafe as well. It can also contribute to the poor health of many other organ tissues.

It is just as bad to have less calcium than is needed. When this occurs, it can lead to an excess of phosphorus. An excess of phosphorus-to-calcium ratio in your bloodstream causes a message to be sent to your body that calcium is needed—and your body will pull that calcium right out of your bones—exactly what most women are worried about.

The only way you can guarantee that you are creating a state of mineral balance in your body at all times is by getting your minerals from a whole food source, where they are naturally balanced by other nutrient cofactors and in amounts small enough to be safely assimilated.

Neither man-made inorganic mineral formulas nor the newer nano-sized mineral products are capable of reproducing the incredible and complex synergy found in any single whole food. Only foods have small, safe amounts of each mineral, so that the body is easily able to quickly utilize each one in harmony with its needs. Eating a variety of whole foods, with the variety of minerals they contain, is ideal.

Essential Nutrients: Amino Acids

Amino acids are the building blocks of protein. Protein molecules make up more than half of the physical structure of most cells and tissues.

Beyond Foods

Proteins are usually thought of as needed for building muscle mass, and this is true; muscle is almost pure protein. Amino acids are needed for far more than muscles, however.

Amino acids also:

- form antibodies to combat invading bacteria and viruses
- are the building blocks of enzymes
- are the building blocks of hormones, which regulate all other body functions
- are essential for carrying oxygen
- are essential in building RNA and DNA, which allows for the correct rebuilding of the genetic code during cellular division

There are ten nonessential amino acids. These, your body can biosynthesize from foods. Then there are ten essential amino acids. You must receive these intact and directly from food sources.

Amino acids do not work as isolates. They always work in concert, often (though not always) in small building blocks called peptides. A *peptide* is created when a small number of amino acids (usually from two to seven) are bound to one or more minerals. Peptides are like Lego building blocks—you can put them together in very large numbers to create something far more complex. I do not recommend isolated amino acid supplements. Using a single amino acid supplement can actually throw off the balance and usefulness of the others present in your diet and body.

There is a common belief that essential amino acids are present only in meat. While it is true that meat offers a concentration of essential amino acids, eating meat comes at a price to your digestion and body energy reserves—which may (or may not) be worthwhile for you.

If you eat meat, I encourage the following guidelines.

Eat only organic, free-range meat. The levels of drugs, steroids, hormones, and other contaminants is extremely high in commercially raised animals, and that is not even considering the quality of life they experience.

Use a variety of meats sources. Most meat contains roughly only 30 to 35 percent of the essential amino acids you need. This means you need to eat a variety of meat in order to have a balance of them all.

Eat smaller portions at each meal. Meat is hard to digest. This is actually a major digestion problem and one most people are not very aware of. I recommend no more than two to four ounces at any single meal.

Here is the analogy I like to use.

Imagine you want a superball to play with, to bounce around the room (imagine you want protein to build muscle mass). Now, eating meat is akin to buying a golf ball and then getting a hacksaw and knife, then cutting away at the incredibly dense outer layers to reach the ball within. It is there—but wow, what a lot of work! And you can only hope you don't lose a finger!

Meat is an incredibly dense, energy-inefficient source of amino acids. Even vegetarian sources can be difficult to digest. (You get advice on making this easier in the section on "Building Block 3: Digestive Nutrients.")

Even when you are eating vegetable proteins (such as beans, nuts, and especially any processed vegetable protein sources like tofu), I recommend you limit intake to no more than three to four ounces in any single meal. You will actually digest your proteins better, meaning you will get more use out of the protein you eat if you eat less at each meal.

You can obtain all your essential amino acids from vegetarian sources in two ways.

1. Eat a variety of protein-rich plant foods that complement one another in amino acid content. Examples include eating corn and beans together, adding mushrooms to any whole grain dish, and including nuts and seeds in a meal.
2. Certain ancient foods are exceptionally rich in amino acid peptides. Peptides are small groups of amino acids bound to minerals. The body uses them like building blocks, creating thousands of different combinations. Other protein rich foods have to be broken down into peptides before the body can use those amino acids. Therefore, peptide-rich ancient foods are valuable, saving your body the energy of digesting heavy proteins.

The two most ancient foods on earth are fungi (mushrooms) and algae. They both offer significant amounts of essential amino acids in smaller peptides. There is one species of edible wild algae that actually contains *all* the essential amino acids in a near-perfect balance for the ideal human profile, as determined by the Food and Nutrition Council.

Without a sufficient, balanced array of all the different amino acids:

- You begin to lose muscle tone.
- You cannot create energy on a cellular level (you will begin to experience fatigue).

- You will begin to lose the ability to create, at will, the complete neurochemical array found in a healthy brain (you may experience brain fog, memory issues, and mood swings).
- You may experience hormone imbalances.

Essential amino acid peptides that are bioavailable (meaning your body can uptake and use them) are truly one of our most essential nutrients!

Essential Nutrients: Essential Fatty Acids

We cannot synthesize essential fatty acids (EFAs) in our body; therefore, we must get them from our diet. Essential fatty acids are the micronutrient components that determine if a fat is a "good fat" or "bad fat."

All EFAs—omega 3s, 6s, 9s, and others—are formed from two truly essential fatty acids: linoleic acid (LA) and alpha-linolenic acid (ALA). These two EFAs form omega 3s and 6s, which are the basis of all other EFA derivatives (omega 9, omega 7, and so on). A healthy body with the right micronutrients can produce all these derivatives.

Once again proving the importance of obtaining nutrients from whole foods or whole-food supplements, your body needs the following five vitamins and minerals in order to convert dietary omega 3s and 6s into the EFA derivatives needed for various life functions.

- vitamins B_3, B_6, and C
- magnesium and zinc

This means that *a deficiency of any of the above five essential nutrients may mimic the degenerative symptoms of an EFA deficiency.*

Beyond Foods

You can find EFAs in oily cold-water fish (such as wild salmon), in some fruits, in seeds and nuts, and in edible algae. It is not essential to take a fish oil supplement. If you wish to take a supplement, most people do well with hemp seed oil or an algae supplement.

If you prefer fish oil, I personally recommend you eat the whole fish, not buy a concentrated oil supplement, because of absorbability problems. There are several studies indicating that fish oil is poorly absorbed.

You also need to consider where the fish was caught. Sadly, many areas of our oceans are severely contaminated. Eating fish from these areas can actually be eating a concentrated serving of heavy metals or other toxins.

EFAs are:

- vital to the flexibility and fluidity of all cells
- required for the normal growth and repair of the skin, blood vessels, and nerve tissues
- essential for healthy nerve and brain function

Essential fatty acids are important for the health of:

- skin
- cognitive function and brain health
- the heart and circulatory system
- hair
- joint mobility

EFAs actively increase the solubility of cholesterol deposits, thereby helping to maintain healthy blood cholesterol levels. They are called "essential" for a reason; recent studies continue to expand our understanding of their importance as micronutrients. For example, one study shows that a lack of EFAs in pregnancy is linked to low birth weight.

One large study, conducted by the Rush Presbyterian St. Luke's Medical Center in Chicago, followed eight hundred participants over several years. The results found that senior citizens who ate one portion of oily fish (a cold-water fish, such as wild salmon) at least once a week were 60 percent less likely to develop Alzheimer's four years later than those who rarely or never ate oily fish.

Essential fatty acids are critical in managing and maintaining a healthy inflammatory response. In fact, it is the balance of omega-3 and omega-6 fatty acids that helps control inflammation. Too much of one or not enough of the other and your body may not be able to respond correctly to disease or even normal metabolic changes. Since chronic inflammation is linked to over three hundred diseases, this is a great example of the essential nature of EFA balance.

Essential Nutrients: Important Phytonutrients

Chlorophyll

> "Chlorophyll is the sun nutrient which is the basis for all plant life activity; the green blood of plants becomes the red blood of animals and humans."
>
> —Philip E. Binzel Jr., MD

In 1912, it was discovered that chlorophyll is very similar to heme, the red pigment in blood responsible for transporting oxygen to all parts of the body.

Heme differs from chlorophyll only by a single central molecule—iron (Fe) in heme and magnesium (Mg) in chlorophyll.

Given the similarity between chlorophyll and heme, it is postulated that the body may be able to directly convert chlorophyll into heme by replacing the central atom. This could improve your oxygen flow and the capacity blood has to oxygenate tissues.

Human Blood Hemoglobin   Plant Chlorophyll

Chlorophyll and Heme from Human Red Blood Cells

There is considerable research and anecdotal evidence that chlorophyll is effective in rebuilding the blood, through metabolic processes that are not yet completely understood.

Chlorophyll assists the body's pH balance. Chlorophyll is both alkalizing and cleansing.

Because of its natural deodorizing ability, chlorophyll has traditionally been used as a mouthwash and gargle. It has been shown to stimulate liver function and excretion of bile, strengthen immunity, and detoxify chemical pollutants. Numerous recent studies also indicate that chlorophyll may have anticarcinogenic and antimutagenic properties.

The highest known concentration of chlorophyll in any food is found in a species of edible wild algae, *Aphanizomenon flos aquae*, or AFA. This dramatic increase of an essential nutrient is a key aspect of wild foods in contrast to farmed foods. The difference in quality and levels of nutrients between wild foods and farmed foods can be profound.

Chlorophyll content per 1 gram

AFA algae *wild*	30 mg
Chlorella *farmed*	28 mg
Spirulina *farmed*	12 mg
Barley grass *farmed*	15 mg
Wheatgrass *farmed*	6 mg

Neuropeptides & Nucleotides

Neuropeptides are the building blocks of *nucleotides*, the protein building blocks RNA and DNA. Having foods rich in the amino acids and amino acid peptides necessary for the production of nucleotides can be a huge nutritional boost to brain and nerve function.

Neuropeptides help to repair, rebuild, and strengthen the neurotransmitters in the brain so that the brain's neurons, or nerve cells, can communicate at peak effectiveness.

Some foods actually contain neuropeptides, and there are studies showing these foods can offer healing benefits.

Beyond Foods

Other Phytonutrients

Phytonutrients are unique chemicals and families of chemicals that come only from plants and have beneficial effects on human and animal health.

There are literally hundreds of phytonutrients. It is estimated that science has identified less than 90 percent of the phytonutrients in plants, and many of those science has identified have been the subject of few if any scientific studies. This is in part because the cost of a study is tremendous. In general, drug companies are the only entities with the money available to afford extensive scientific studies. It is a fact that all drug companies are for profit. The studies they fund are focused on drugs, which are huge sources of monetary gain.

There are studies done on phytonutrients via government grants, but sadly they are often underfunded. This is actually one reason you don't see more studies on the powerful benefits of food-based nutrients—there simply is not enough money to be made from them.

In fact, drug companies sometimes fund studies in hopes of disproving benefits from food-based nutrients. And studies that find otherwise might not be published.

A very few of the phytonutrient families we know are beneficial include:

- beta glucans (complex sugar molecules)
- flavonoids
- polyphenols
- catechins

Beta glucans are incredibly powerful complex sugar molecules. They have been proven, over decades of research, to support innate immune function. They don't stimulate the immune system; they help it to respond appropriately and powerfully. They are found in several foods. The strongest for human health benefits are the beta glucans found in mushrooms and other fungi.

Flavonoids, polyphenols, and catechins are found in dozens of foods, including grape skins, tea leaves, many fruits and vegetables, and tonic mushrooms. They are each entire families of antioxidants. They also show a wide variety of other important benefits. The reasons for these varied benefits are not completely understood. Examples of the benefits beyond being antioxidants include reducing cardiovascular disease, reducing tooth decay, supporting healthy liver function, and much more.

Most phytochemical compounds are considered nonessential. However, science is proving they are an important part of the human diet and health. It is important to remember that less than 10 percent of phytochemicals have been identified. In addition to acting as antioxidants, other phytonutrients may have anticarcinogenic effects and beneficial effects on chronic inflammation and immune function support. It is clear that eating phytonutrients properly and in moderation can play a positive role in human health.

Summary

A *superfood* is a whole food that acts as powerhouse of concentrated nutrients, offering a lot of micronutrient nutrition for comparatively few calories.

Micronutrients are "the rest of the story" about nutrition. A micronutrient is a substance that is essential in minute amounts for the proper growth and metabolism of a living organism.

Beyond Foods

Micronutrients include trace minerals, vitamins, and co-vitamins. In addition, superfoods may also have essential fatty acids (EFAs) and essential amino acids, as well as other phytonutrients, such as pigments, food-based antioxidants, and a host of other molecules only now being recognized as beneficial.

Many people are starving for micronutrients, which can lead to physical, mental, and emotional problems.

What You Can Do

Add any of the following nutrient-packed foods for a simple upgrade to any diet.

- Eat sprouted and organic multigrain breads and cereals instead of processed white or wheat. This is a good way to get a variety of sprouted grains into anyone and simpler than sprouting your own. It is vital that you buy organic because nonorganic grain is potentially GMO.
- Use organic nut butters (like almond) on your toast instead of any type of margarine spread.
- Shop the perimeter of your store. In general, this is where most whole foods will be found, such as produce, a meat counter, and bulk whole foods like grains and nuts.
- Use organic rice, nut, or grain milk. Pasteurized dairy is not digestible. Soy is also hard to digest, and unless it is organic, it will be GMO.
- Go to your local grower's market and buy local organic vegetables and fruits. You may even find local organically raised meats. Local farmers and your body will thank you!
- Sprouts are the seeds of legumes, grains, and nuts that have been germinated into baby plants within three to five days. Specifically, sprouts contain a high concentration of antioxidant

nutrients, such as vitamins A, C, E, and B-complex. Sprouts often contain trace minerals, including much-needed selenium and zinc, plus bioflavonoids as well as chlorophyll and fiber. Health gurus have been promoting these powerhouses for decades. Many grocers now carry organic sprouts, including alfalfa, broccoli, kale, and sunflower. Buy local and organic or learn to sprout your own.

You can eat the next two foods as cooked grains.

- Millet is high in iron, magnesium, potassium, silicon, B vitamins, and vitamin E.
- Quinoa is an ancient grain that provides a more usable protein than meat. It is a rich source of minerals, including calcium, which is in a form more assimilable than that found in milk.
- Parsley, cilantro, and other fresh culinary herbs, such as rosemary and oregano, are all nutrient powerhouses. Nutrients found in herbs can include high levels of beta-carotene, vitamin B_{12}, chlorophyll, calcium, vitamin C, and other beneficial nutrients.

Wild Foods

In Traditional Chinese Medicine (TCM), the nutrients in wild foods are considered up to eight hundred times more potent than farmed foods. This is because a wild food has to continually adapt to survive its environment. Those adaptive qualities become adaptogenic nutrients, which can benefit us.

Is there proof of the value of wild-grown foods versus commercially farmed foods? Are wild-grown foods really better for you, stronger, more viable, and more nutrient rich than farmed foods?

Beyond Foods

The following examples affirm that wild foods offer benefits that help the healing and vitality of your body.

Professor Katharine Milton of the University of California, Berkeley, studied wild monkeys in Panama and found that the wild fruits, flowers, and plants that the monkeys ate contained far more nutrients than the typical diet of humans. This included higher levels of calcium, potassium, and other micronutrients. The wild fruits also have a different sugar content than farmed fruits.

The next example of the value of wild foods is from *Let's Live* magazine. They compared three nutritional factors between wild and farmed Atlantic salmon.

Per serving, farmed salmon had 10.5 grams of fat, 175 calories, and 52 milligrams of sodium. The wild salmon had nearly 30 percent less fat, fewer calories, and less sodium for the same serving!

The major differences between the two foods include:

- Farmed salmon are penned and fed commercially manufactured foods, along with antibiotics and growth hormones.
- Wild salmon must find the foods it needs and survive in a harsh and unpredictable environment.

Lastly, a study done through the University of North Carolina in 2014 details the process of how wild berries develop health-protective phytochemicals to thrive in the wild. Edible berries then offer broad-spectrum health benefits to animals via these phytonutrients.

The following is a list of wild foods fairly easy to add to your diet. Although many of the foods below are now farmed, this has occurred in just in the last few decades. These foods are ancient foods, tens of thousands of years older than most farmed fruits or vegetables. All have many powerful nutrients developed from surviving in the wild for millennia.

Quality control is absolutely paramount when adding any wild superfood. I recommend you only use those which are certified organic from a reliable certification agency. Also look for products which offer other third party validation of safety and quality, such as an NSF or wild-crafted certification.

- Wild microalgae— There are a few edible species of edible microalgae. These algae have thousands of years of use in cultures around the world. Farmed microalgae which you can find in supplements include the green algae chlorella, red sea algae *dunaliella salina* and two edible bluegreen microalga. The most commonly available bluegreen algae is spirulina. There is one truly wild microalgae, *Aphanizomenon flos aquae*, or AFA. It is wild-harvested in a natural freshwater ecosystem. AFA has had hundreds of different studies showing a myriad of benefits. All microalgae are helpful for people who aren't absorbing nutrients properly; AFA has a greater than 95 percent assimilation rate.
- Wild sea vegetables or seaweeds are macro-algae. Like microalgae, they provide a highly digestible source of all minerals, including those that are very scarce in the Western diet. Sea vegetables alkalinize the blood, and some are proven to remove toxic metals, another important benefit. Some sea vegetables have been shown to markedly reduce cholesterol levels. Easiest to find are dulse, wakame, kombu, and nori. These can be added to salads and soups. Others, such as bladderwrack and *Eklonia cava*, can be found in supplements.
- Tonic mushrooms—These are mushrooms proven to be loaded with adaptogenic nutrients. Like the microalgae, some are now

cultivated but retain many of their nutrients from growing wild for thousands of years. Like algae, tonic mushrooms have been used to great benefit in cultures around the world. Shitake and maitake are delicious and found in the produce aisle. Recommended wild mushrooms include morels, chanterelles, and black trumpet. Tonic mushroom with a wide variety of proven and powerful benefits found in supplements include reishi, *Poria cocos*, and lion's mane.

Note: do not harvest your own mushrooms unless and until you have been educated on safe species found in your area.

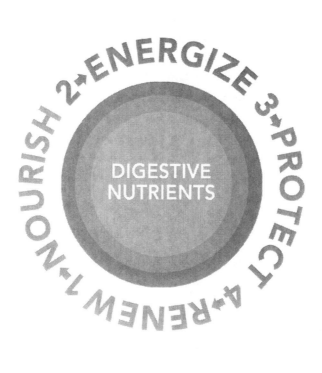

Chapter 6
Building Block 2: Digestive Nutrients

Digestion is much more than getting calories from your food. Digestion is truly the basis for health itself. Without the ability to absorb and then assimilate nutrients from the foods we eat, good health is not possible.

How well (or poorly) your digestive system works directly impacts immune function and liver health. Your immune system determines how you are able to live in the world around you, including whether you are adequately protected against invaders or if your body goes on a rampage and attacks itself. Cancers and autoimmune disorders have a link to poor gut health and the resulting poor immune function.

Beyond Foods

The liver is responsible for maintaining a clean house. Millions of dead cells and other toxic residues of metabolism have to be cleared on a daily basis, and a healthy liver is essential for this process.

Digestive nutrients help your body break down foods into usable nutrients. Your body must take large food molecules and convert them into smaller nutrients that can be safely absorbed into your bloodstream. It takes less energy to turn food into fuel for your cells when digestive nutrients are present. The energy saved translates into vitality—an energy and enjoyment of life.

Digestive nutrients include good bacteria—probiotics—and food enzymes.

Digestive Nutrients in History

All traditional cultures around the world have fermented or cultured foods. These are live foods, naturally rich in digestive nutrients—good bacteria and enzymes. Tempeh, miso, yogurt, aged cheeses, raw vinegar, sauerkraut, kimchee, pickles, kombucha, and even raw ales are all traditional fermented foods. Fermentation was a way to safely preserve foods before refrigeration was available. These foods were eaten daily, some more often during certain seasons, and helped humans survive in times when nutrition was less than optimal—long winters and early spring in particular.

When prepared according to tradition and consumed raw, fermented foods give us powerful and proven health benefits, including immune function support and optimized digestion. However, in industrialized nations, most fermented foods are heated, sterilized, and processed or pasteurized and no longer offer any digestive benefits.

Enzymes

An enzyme is a molecule that acts as a catalyst. When an enzyme is present, other molecules are able to change without harmful effects, while the enzyme itself is not affected.

Enzymes, quite literally, allow life as we know it, to exist. They allow the chemical actions and reactions that create life to occur at a vastly quicker pace—up to a million times faster than would be possible without the enzyme. Without enzymes, each chemical reaction within our body would happen so slowly that life (as we know it) wouldn't be possible. The chemistry involved in having a thought could take days or weeks instead of a millisecond!

Imagine reactions happening as slowly as a crystal grows in the earth; that is the difference that enzymes make. For this reason, science actually defines life by the presence of enzymes.

All bodily functions and the production of energy to fuel these functions are dependent upon specific enzymes. Researchers have identified over 2,700 enzymes in the human body—and they are still counting. Each one produces one type, and only one type, of chemical reaction. As amazing as it seems, the absence of a single type of enzyme can cause death. Many profound genetic disorders involve mistakes in genetic coding for a single enzymatic function.

Enzymes are one of the most studied elements of the human body, yet most doctors do not know the incredible value of plant-based enzyme supplements.

According to Dr. Anthony J. Cichoke in *Enzymes and Enzyme Therapy*, "Without them, many of the body's chemical reactions would never take place. Without enzymes, there would be no breathing, no digestion, no growth, no blood coagulation, no perception of the senses, and no reproduction. Our bodies contain millions of enzymes, which continually renew, maintain, and protect us. No person, plant, or animal could exist without them."

In every body, there is ongoing competition for the raw materials needed to create enzymes. We need essential amino acids and minerals, as well as energy, in order to create an enzyme. Different enzymes are needed for correct digestion, immune system support, energy production, and good metabolism.

Your body uses enzymes to safely create the cellular energy that fuels your daily activities. Therefore, daily you need the required nutrients to replace these enzymes. With an optimal diet, you may have enough raw materials (essential amino acids, minerals, and energy) in order to create enough enzymes for good health. However, nearly everyone is lacking enough enzymes to correctly digest their food. The truth is for thousands of years, humans have been dependent on fermented foods to help provide missing digestive enzymes—and most modern diets no longer have them.

Digestive Needs

When food is not fully digested, it sits in our intestines and becomes toxic residue. Whether dietary or environmental, toxins require the immune system to remove them through the action of enzymes.

Therefore, the more incompletely digested food we have in our system, the more enzymes our immune system needs to deal with the resulting toxins and debris. This in turn leaves less raw material to create the enzymes available for correct digestion; it becomes a vicious cycle.

Food enzymes are digestive nutrients that have the ability to promote correct digestion, beginning in the stomach. This is desperately needed because people in America are in the midst of a health crisis—*indigestion*.

- Nearly 10 percent of Americans—nearly thirty million people—experience indigestion and heartburn daily.
- An estimated sixty to ninety million Americans experience indigestion at least once a week.
- Indigestion or heartburn costs our economy over two billion dollars *a week*.
- Studies show that people who suffer from indigestion have impaired social, emotional, and physical functioning.

The bottom line is chronic indigestion has a profound impact on daily living.

How often do you sit down to enjoy a leisurely meal—freshly prepared from fresh, local organic vegetables and meats, free of added preservatives, fillers, or colorants? A meal that has no time limit?

Indigestion can be the result of eating too much or too fast. It can be caused by eating when we are overtired or under stress or when we eat foods that are greasy, fatty, or processed. Indigestion also occurs when we do not have time to relax and allow our body the energy and time necessary to digest our meal.

Digestion begins in the mouth. Chewing breaks our food into small pieces and mixes food with the first important enzymes, which are found in saliva. These salivary enzymes begin the chemical breakdown of carbohydrates.

Beyond Foods

So, what happens if you do not chew your food well? Or if you eat so fast that not enough saliva is produced? Even if you make an effort to chew correctly, low enzyme count in saliva is a common problem, especially as you age.

Since the next step in digestion is the stomach, that is where any problems will land—literally. A lack of proper chewing can lead to the improper digestion of carbohydrates, which is a major cause of acid stomach. Why does this happen?

Our body understands that if food cannot be broken down correctly in the stomach, it will not be completely and safely absorbed or assimilated in the intestines. *Therefore, whenever we need a boost to digestion, more stomach acid is produced.*

The body responds to under-chewing, overeating, stress, and fatty, oily, or processed foods by attempting to strengthen the digestive process. Therefore, one of the side effects of a poor diet or poor eating habits is an increase in the production of stomach acid *because* ...

Stomach acid is essential for correct digestion!

- Stomach acid breaks down otherwise indigestible protein bonds.
- Stomach acid is essential in order to retrieve minerals from our food.
- Stomach acid signals the pancreas to release enzymes that are essential for digestion in the intestines.
- Stomach acid kills many pathogenic bacteria and so is considered a part of our innate immune system's defense against disease.

Today, antacids are the second leading over-the-counter (OTC) medication sold—nearly four billion dollars in sales in 2014. Since antacids work by absorbing stomach acid, *they do nothing* to help the actual digestive process. Instead, they merely take away the pain, which is an essential symptom to warn us that digestion is not occurring.

Antacids also have some nasty side effects.

- calcium salts antacids: constipation, bloating, cramps, kidney stones, and kidney disease
- sodium salts antacids: not for use if you are on a salt-restricted diet or have heart disease or suspected heart disease
- magnesium salts antacids: may cause diarrhea, can lower blood pressure sufficiently to cause heartbeat irregularities, can cause central nervous system difficulties
- aluminum salts antacids: are linked to osteoporosis and should be avoided by women after menopause
- most: interference with the body's ability to assimilate vitamin B_{12}
- all: potential for constipation

It is not uncommon to find that people who get chronic bacterial infections also regularly use an antacid—a drug that prevents the stomach from fulfilling its role in immune function.

Plant-Based Digestive Enzymes

One way to get more enzymes in your diet is to eat enough fresh raw foods daily. Dr. Ted Morter, in his book *Health and Wellness*, says that 70 to 80 percent of our diet should be made up of raw foods to help supply the body's enzymatic needs.

Beyond Foods

Most of us do not eat a diet with 70 percent raw foods daily. Many people eat a bit of raw fruit, often only seasonally, and maybe a side of salad with dinner, but that's not even close to the recommended daily raw food intake. Americans are accustomed to eating mainly cooked foods, which contain no enzymes. There are no enzymes because when foods are cooked or processed, enzymes are rendered inactive.

Even when foods are raw, they may not have sufficient enzymes.

If produce is not organic, the enzymes will have been compromised by the use of chemicals. In agribusiness farming, many raw foods are harvested weeks or even months before you buy them. We now have a world marketplace, and nearly all imported produce is irradiated, which destroys enzymes.

It is best to eat from your local growers' market. Even then, if produce is more than a few days old, the enzymes begin to break down because enzymes in fresh foods last a few days at the most. Historically, many foods would be fermented to aid in their preservation. Fermentation is a process using good bacteria, and enzymes are a by-product of living fermented foods. Unfortunately, today most fermented foods are rendered enzymeless through pasteurization or other sterilization processes.

Therefore, it is my opinion that adding a food-based digestive enzyme is one of the best ways to help ensure health and vitality. With most modern diets, enzyme supplements are essential in order to digest and assimilate nutrients in our foods.

Enzyme Supplement Benefits

When you add an acid-stable food enzyme to your meal, your body requires less acid to break down food in preparation for entering the intestines. This enzyme will not only aid the body's process of digestion by breaking food down into absorbable nutrients; it can potentially lessen your chance of dealing with acid indigestion.

Leaky-gut syndrome is rampant. It occurs when partially digested food molecules—in particular, complex proteins—leak out through the lining of your gut into the bloodstream. As they roam throughout the body, these large complex food molecules stimulate your immune system. This can eventually lead to an overactive immune response. This is one way in which incorrect digestion, over time, can also lead to other health issues.

So while digestive enzyme supplements are primarily used to support healthy digestion, enzyme use can help maintain vibrant health on every level and in every system in the human body. Our need for enzymes is hard science and a major part of our physiology.

An example of how dependent digestion is on enzymes occurs with vitamin A. When you eat beta-carotene (which is the food precursor to vitamin A), an enzyme in the intestines turns it into vitamin A (retinal). No enzymes—no vitamin A from beta-carotene.

Food enzymes can be grown on a fungal medium; isolated from pineapples, papayas, and a few other fruits; and derived from an animal pancreas, usually bovine or porcine. Neither fruit nor animal-source enzymes are very effective for human use.

Issues with fruit and animal source enzymes include the following.

- With pancreatic enzymes, there is no telling the health status of the animal used.
- Animal and fruit enzymes are primarily only proteases—which means they only help with the digestion of proteins.

- Animal and fruit enzymes work in a very narrow pH range.
- Animal and fruit enzymes work on a very narrow range of protein types.

The most effective enzymes are those grown on a fungal medium, typically *Aspergillus orzyae*. This process is safe—*there is no fungus present in the enzymes thus created*. This process can be used to create an effective broad spectrum of plant-based enzymes. These enzymes function and are able to be active in a very wide pH range—from 2 to 12—and you can find formulas that literally digest nearly every type of food you may eat. The most effective formulas will contain many of the following enzymes.

- a variety of protease enzymes—There are several different types; each breaks down a specific type of large protein molecule into smaller amino-acid peptide groups.
- a variety of amylase enzymes—Again, there is more than one type; each breaks down one type of carbohydrate into much more digestible simple and complex sugars. They also help release the other nutrients found in the carbohydrate (such as vitamins and antioxidants). There are several types of nutrients found in carbohydrates, but if your body is not breaking them down effectively, you may not be absorbing those important nutrients.
- lipase enzymes break down large fat molecules into essential fatty acids and other fatty acids (which are much more easily digested).
- miscellaneous other enzymes, including those that help break down milk, blood, and specific types of sugars

Enzymes require minerals as cofactors. Therefore, an enzyme formula that is microblended with a mineral-rich whole food, such as algae, offers a powerful increase in enzyme activity and potency.

Enzymes can provide a nearly miraculous enhancement of the digestion of cooked or processed meals. Benefits of using food-based digestive enzymes include:

- less bloating
- less or no gas
- reduced excess acid
- reduced or decreased tiredness after eating
- reduced food sensitivities and reactions

Digestive Nutrients: Probiotics

Probiotics (from the Latin, "for life") refers to the beneficial bacteria with which humans have developed symbiotic relationships.

We always have bacteria in our bodies—a *lot* of bacteria. If you were to put together all the DNA in your body, less than 10 percent will be DNA from *you*. This means that over 90 percent of the DNA in your body is bacterial in origin.

Probiotic bacteria have been proven to affect human DNA and appear to have the ability to help turn on—or turn off—the genetic propensity for some diseases.

Thus, the question is not: "Are there bacteria in my gut?" The question is: "Do I have good bacteria supporting my health and DNA, or do I have bacteria fighting the health of my body and DNA?"

Having healthy microbes in the gut is shown to help:

- maintain a healthy weight
- increase a healthy immune response to bacteria and viruses
- reduce inflammation

Beyond Foods

Today, probiotics are finally being recognized by the medical establishment as a very important supplement to consume daily, not just for help with health issues, but also for keeping healthy in a stress-filled lifestyle. Dr. Oz mentioned the importance of probiotics on his show, and CNN had a segment on probiotics recently. Just about everywhere, another doctor is referring to the importance of probiotics.

The following represent summaries of only a few of the many dozens of recent probiotics research studies. These are direct excerpts from the *Clinical Applications of Probiotics in Human Health* symposium, which took place in 2007 at the University of Nevada School of Medicine. The symposium provided attendees with cutting-edge information on the use of probiotics to enhance health.

The summaries discuss the beneficial results from using probiotics supplements for many degenerative conditions.

These statements are being made by researchers and MDs.

> Dr. McFarland reviewed data from 216 clinical trials of probiotics in health conditions ranging from antibiotic-associated diarrhea to allergies and eczema. She also reviewed highly positive data for the use of both certain types of acidophilus and multispecies probiotics in a variety of clinical conditions, including the prevention of antibiotic-associated diarrhea and reduction of the risk of pediatric allergic diseases.
>
> Dr. Jose Saavedra, associate professor of pediatrics at Johns Hopkins University School of Medicine and a pioneer in pediatric probiotic research, gave data on the importance of the intestinal microbiota for immune

system maturation and modulation and the role of bad bacteria in the current epidemic of childhood allergic diseases. He highlighted the importance of *Bifidobacterium* to improve immune function and enhance gut maturation in...preterm infants and enhance innate immunity...in adults.

Dr. David Traver, a pediatrician specializing in the biomedical treatment of children with autism-spectrum disorders noted that poor gut barrier function is common and well-documented in these children and that...incompletely digested casein (milk products) and gluten (wheat products) may significantly contribute to the poor nerve function manifestations of autism. Dr. Traver presented data showing that exposure to broad-spectrum antibiotics may be a trigger in the development of autism...and that probiotics have become a cornerstone in the biomedical treatment of autistic spectrum disorders.

Dr. Stig Bengmark, chief of surgery for over 20 years at Lund University Hospital in Sweden, stated that his research interest in probiotics began in 1986 when he and colleagues reviewed the incidence of infections in their patients undergoing liver resection and found that all the postoperative infections occurred in those treated with antibiotics and no infections developed in patients who had not received antibiotics. He speculated that many of the chronic diseases now prevalent in industrial societies are related to lack of dietary consumption of important probiotic species.

Dr. Philippe Marteau, world-renowned authority on the use of probiotics in inflammatory bowel disease, presented clinical data demonstrating the clinical efficacy of a probiotic formulation containing eight species for the management of ulcerative colitis and pouchitis, a complication of the surgical management of ulcerative colitis; and Crohn's disease.

The Gut and Your Brain

Most people don't realize the gut isn't just where we absorb nutrients. As Dr. Stephen Holt, MD, author of *Natural Ways to Digestive Health*, states, your gut is actually and effectively acting as a second brain. *The digestive nervous system contains as many neurons as the spinal cord.*

It is an interesting fact that the greatest concentration and production of serotonin, which is involved in mood control, depression, and behavior changes, is found in the intestines, not the brain.

A study published recently in the medical journal *Neurogastroenterology & Motility* found that mice that lacked good gut bacteria behaved differently from normal mice, engaging in what would be referred to as high-risk behavior. This changed behavior was accompanied by neurochemical changes in the mice's brains.

This may explain why researchers keep finding that depression, fear, and a variety of mood-related problems may be linked to an imbalance of bacteria in the gut. Many people with poor gut health also have symptoms of constipation, allergies, bloating, fungus on toenails, and more.

Your Gut and Immune Function

Our gastrointestinal (GI) tract is an immune hub. Seventy percent of our immune activity occurs in our GI tract. About 80 percent of your body's protective immunoglobulins are produced there.

A hyper, weak, or confused immune system is often found along with an unhealthy bacterial overload in the gut. Bad bacteria will leave your gut deficient of many ingredients that help keep the immune system in balance. Your innate immune system interacts with and is dependent on the microbes in your gut. If they are probiotics—the "good guys"—your immune and nerve functions are supported. If they are hostile, you are basically under continual attack.

Almost all degenerative conditions fall into one of three categories of immune system malfunction.

1. The immune system is weakened, and the result is called an immune suppression disease. Examples include cancer and AIDS.
2. The immune system overreacts to stress and other normally benign factors and becomes hyper-responsive to normal stimuli. Examples include asthma, eczema, and allergies.
3. A malfunctioning or confused immune system causes autoimmune reactions (autoimmune diseases) where antibodies target the body's own tissues. Examples include rheumatoid arthritis, MS, and lupus.

When dealing with any degenerative condition, one should work toward balancing the immune system, and this is where the role of probiotics becomes of the utmost importance.

Beyond Foods

The highest source of contamination in the body, other than a cut in the skin, is the food you eat. Probiotic bacteria are the body's second line of defense against microbes, fungi, and bad bacteria (after stomach acid). Over millennia, the human body has created a symbiotic relationship with hundreds of species of good bacteria. They colonize our gut as colonies and then produce chemicals that protect them, and us, from bad bacteria that may be ingested.

In return for protecting us from bacterial, fungal, and microbial invaders, the good bacteria get a small portion of the nutrients we ingest.

Our relationship and dependency on good bacteria begins at birth. When born via natural vaginal birth with a healthy mother, the newborn's skin is literally inoculated with about seventeen species of beneficial bacteria. These proceed to inhabit the skin where they gently wake up the child's skin-based immune system and condition the infant to his or her new life in an open world. When an infant is breastfed, he or she ingests a specific type of *bifidum* bacteria from the mother's milk, which gently supports the newborn's gut immune function.

In the United States today, 30 percent of births are via C-section. More and more, it is becoming routine to give mothers antibiotics right after birth, even if they are not ill. This practice can set our children up with immune deficiencies from birth because of the lack of healthy gut bacteria.

Some studies find that babies born by C-section, deprived of their mother's vaginal probiotics during birth, have a higher risk of celiac disease, type 1 diabetes, and obesity. Early-life use of antibiotics—which tear through microbial ecosystems like a typhoon—has also been linked to allergies, inflammatory bowel disease, and obesity.

There are hundreds of species of probiotic bacteria that are transient. These are bacteria that come in briefly and then leave, never actually living in our gut for any space of time. However, they appear to play an important role in supporting the health of our permanent colonizing bacteria.

There are at least eight to ten species of good bacteria, which we need to colonize our gut permanently.

Science isn't always consistent about what, exactly, goes wrong with our probiotic microbes in disease situations. But a recurrent theme is that loss of diversity—fewer species of the "good guys"—correlates with the emergence of illness.

Items that harm probiotic colonies include chlorinated water, caffeine, carbonated beverages, drugs, antibiotics, and stress hormones.

How Probiotics Work

Probiotics help support healthy immune function and good intestinal barrier function (by only allowing completely digested nutrients through the intestinal wall into our bloodstream). A newer study shows probiotics also help prevent the production of the biochemicals involved in allergic responses (called cytokines). This is an important study, as it was discovered that the probiotics had more effect in people who were healthy than in those already ill with allergies.

This really points to the benefits of maintaining your health and gut flora. There is solid evidence that probiotic DNA interacts with ours. We are vulnerable to our gut bacteria—good or bad—on a genetic level.

There are two main families of bacteria that are absolutely essential:

- Acidophilus family—in general, this bacteria family inhabits the upper GI tract (small intestines).
- Bifidus family—in general, this bacteria family colonizes the lower GI tract (large intestines).

Acidophilus

Acidophilus works with the immune cells in the intestinal tract (called Peyer's patches). These little packets of immune cells are a part of our lymph system and depend on acidophilus to function correctly. Immune cells in the gut comprise about 70 to 75 percent of the immune system with which we are born (the other 25 to 30 percent are in the skin). Our innate immune cells work closely with acidophilus colonies.

Acidophilus has been shown to actually help mitigate DNA damage from cadmium exposure, showing that the presence of these bacteria offers protective action against heavy-metal toxicity.

There are two hundred different strains of *Lactobacillus acidophilus*, some thirteen of which have quite strong antibiotic qualities.

There are several acidophilus strains marketed as "the best." That's because it is fairly simple to create a new strain of bacteria; they mutate easily. At that point, they can be patented by the manufacturer, who then literally "owns" that strain and who of course now wants to make some money from their investment. A quick study with a few people and *voila*! There is a new proven "best" strain of acidophilus.

Based on decades of long-term research done on probiotics, it is my opinion that the most beneficial strain of acidophilus is DDS-1. It has been widely researched and its abilities to support human health documented by renowned expert scientists, such as Dr. Khem Shahani at the University of Nebraska.

DDS-1 has powerful anticarcinogenic properties and produces effective natural antibiotic substances that have been shown to potentially deactivate eleven known disease-causing bacteria.

Bifidus

Bifidus bacteria are the primary colonizers in our large intestine. They help us absorb and then assimilate bioactive vitamin B_{12}. Bifidus is essential for finishing the digestive process. It helps to prevent toxins from building up in the colon and supports regular elimination. Bifidus bacteria are an essential component of the natural ongoing cleansing process, helping to eliminate toxic buildup.

In what I feel is groundbreaking research, bifidus has been shown to have a profound effect on the physical and emotional well-being of children. Evidence suggests that the bifidus bacterium:

- provides immune protection for the first 1.5 years of life after birth
- prevents and eases symptoms of colic in infants
- provides a sense of well-being and even self-esteem
- provides a sense of nourishment, thus helping to maintain healthy weight

Bifidus also has shown positive effects on sleep in adults.

Summary

Digestion is much more than eating for energy. Digestion is truly the basis for health itself. Without the ability to absorb and utilize the nutrients found in the foods we eat, good health is not possible.

Beyond Foods

Digestive nutrients help your body to correctly break down foods into usable elements. When food is more effectively absorbed into your blood, it takes less energy for your body to turn it into fuel for your cells.

Digestive nutrients include beneficial bacteria—probiotics—and food enzymes.

Plant-based digestive enzymes are molecules that help to break down proteins, fats, and carbohydrates into usable nutrients. Foods that are cooked, preserved, or packaged are very difficult for our body to break down completely. By breaking down food into molecules that are able to be correctly absorbed into the bloodstream, enzymes ensure that our food can be effectively assimilated.

Probiotics are needed for proper digestion and correct immune function. Probiotics help inhibit the overgrowth of other bacteria that can be dangerous. They are also needed to produce B-vitamin complexes. These friendly bacteria are essential for a healthy nervous system and can even affect the health of our DNA.

What You Can Do

Here are some easy steps you can take to help increase the amount of probiotics and enzymes in your diet.

- Eat lots of fresh raw vegetables and fruits. When fresh enough, they are filled with natural food enzymes. Organic is always preferable. Best is local and organic.
- Add organic, non-GMO miso to your meals. This is a healthful fermented soy paste you can use to flavor salad dressings and other dishes. Be sure not to overheat it, or you will destroy the beneficial bacteria and enzymes.

- Eat live-culture fermented foods. Kombucha, live-culture yogurt, and raw sauerkraut are examples you might find locally made.
- Eat only raw (aged or sharp) organic cheese. This healthier option contains good bacteria and enzymes and is a more digestible form of dairy than milk or other cheeses. The ingredients may include "cultured milk."
- Get a good water filter for drinking and cooking. This helps preserve the good bacteria in your gut. Even a faucet filter is helpful.
- Because eating enough raw foods can be difficult, use a good probiotic and plant-based enzyme supplement.

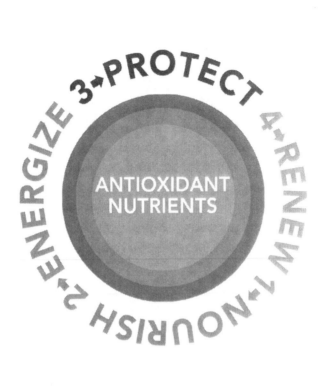

Chapter 7
Building Block 3: Antioxidants to Protect Cellular Function

An *antioxidant* is a molecule that is able to safely neutralize free radicals. *Free radicals* are molecules that are unbalanced at a molecular level. They attempt to rebalance their molecule by stealing an electron. They can attack your blood and cells anywhere in your body.

ROS Free Radicals

Reactive Oxygen Species

There are several kinds of free radicals, but the ones that cause us the most problems are the *oxygen free radicals*, also called reactive oxygen species (ROS). ROS free radicals are especially unstable and aggressive. In an attempt to rebalance, they either bind or scavenge electrons from other molecules—which are in our living cells. This scavenging process often results in a cascade of cellular damage.

The ROS free radical begins as a simple free radical form and then changes into other free radicals during a destructive series of interactions with our cells. This cycle is called the *inflammation cascade*, named for the terrible result these free radicals have in our body.

In this cascade, each new free radical formed is more destructive than the one before it. Each free radical in this chain is different in chemical structure and affects a different part of the cell it is attacking.

It might be compared to falling down a flight of stairs. You trip on one step and are bruised; you stumble down two steps and sprain an ankle; you fall down the whole flight and wind up in the hospital.

In this chain of changing ROS free radicals, each one will be neutralized only by certain antioxidants. This is a very important concept to remember. Most antioxidants are able to neutralize only some of the specific free radicals within this chain of destructive ROS free radicals—but not all of them.

By eating a variety of antioxidants, we ensure that we can neutralize a variety of these destructive ROS free radicals and protect our cells from the ultimate damage, which is mutation to cellular DNA (a major factor in the development of cancer).

Steps in the Oxygen Free Radical Cascade

Singlet oxygen—This begins the cascade of ROS damage to cells. It forms from the molecules of oxygen you breathe and is impossible to avoid. Also triggered by ultraviolet light, singlet oxygen targets tissue and cell components, causing structural changes. It initiates the formation of enzymes that destroy elastin and collagen. This damage is particularly noticeable in skin as dark spots, wrinkles and other signs of sun damage and aging.

Damage Caused: decreased blood supply to cells

Neutralized by: coenzyme Q10 and carotenoid pigments (such as beta-carotene)

Superoxide—This free radical is generated in mitochondria (the energy factories within every cell), in the cardiovascular system, and more. This inflammatory agent attacks cells and interrupts blood flow and other cellular functions. It also destroys enzymes and cell membranes, leaving the cell vulnerable.

Damage caused: lessened nutrient exchange in cells, lesser ability to remove cellular toxins

Neutralized by: superoxide dismutase (SOD); vitamins C and E; the minerals selenium, zinc, copper, and manganese; and coenzyme Q10.

Lipid peroxyl—This ROS free radical continues cell destruction by hardening and deforming lipids (fats) in cell walls and in intercellular fluids, leaving cell walls weak and unable to function.

Damage caused: poor cellular function, weakened ability to repair

Neutralized by: coenzyme Q10, vitamin E

Hydrogen peroxide—Although not a direct free radical, it is dangerous because it easily crosses the cell membrane and enters the nucleus, hardening and deforming protein molecules. Worse, it converts to the hydroxyl radical (see following) in the presence of iron.

Damage caused: poor immune system response, slower actions and reactions on the cellular level

Neutralized by: glutathione peroxidase, catalase

Hydroxyl radical—The most dangerous of the oxygen free radicals, it can attack and mutate DNA. Usually not salvageable, the target cell is destroyed by the body's immune system. This radical can be prevented by eliminating the preceding free radicals.

Damage caused: DNA mutation

Neutralized by: superoxide dismutase, cellular death

There are several sources of ROS free radicals in daily life. Common ones include:

- pollution
- tap water
- herbicides, pesticides, and other contaminants in nonorganic foods
- drugs
- bacteria
- stress

Beyond Foods

Highly processed foods, trans fats, and refined sugar are also implicated as major sources of free radical production, as is a diet lacking essential vitamins and nutrients to help our bodies produce antioxidants to fight free radical damage.

Intense exercise can also lead to excess free radical production, because they are a by-product of cellular energy metabolism. The more you work out your muscles and use energy, the more free radicals are produced as a result.

ROS free radicals are implicated in over three hundred different diseases and chronic conditions because they contribute to a physical process known as *oxidative stress*.

Oxidative Stress

Oxygen is necessary for life as we know it. We need it to breathe, to release energy when we eat, and for almost every single chemical action in our body. However, it is the nature of oxygen to form oxygen free radicals (ROS) as a by-product of these metabolic actions.

Our bodies actually use some of these free radicals. Our white blood cells use them to destroy invaders, and our liver needs them for some of its detoxifying functions. In a healthy body that is young and not overly stressed, our body has plenty of antioxidants, both circulating in our blood and within each cell, to neutralize free radicals.

When we experience stressors in our bodies and lives and if our diet doesn't provide antioxidants, we may begin to produce more ROS free radicals than we can easily neutralize.

According to the *Theory of Oxidative Stress*, we age because of the accumulation of damage done by free radicals. The process that creates this accumulated damage is called oxidative stress (OS). OS accelerates aging because of *chronic inflammation.*

Inflammation is a natural and essential part of the healing process. When you are injured—for example, by a fall, a burn, or free radical damage to a cell—inflammatory signals are sent out. These signals mobilize immune cells and healing support to the injured area.

Chronic inflammation occurs when those chemical signals aren't able to mobilize the appropriate healing response and immune help. Through chronic inflammation, OS first causes damage to cells and then to entire organ systems.

Antioxidants

Antioxidants are an essential part of how our bodies cope with the environmental pollution that surrounds us, inside and out.

Antioxidants neutralize free radicals and protect cells from oxidative stress injury caused by environmental toxins. They help our body recover from toxic damage resulting from metabolic waste.

Antioxidants are essential for healthy immune function. They can either be made in the body or assimilated from the diet.

Enzyme (Innate) Antioxidants

The body makes *enzyme antioxidants.* These are complex proteins that often incorporate microminerals, such as selenium or zinc, in their intricate structures. Because innate antioxidants can neutralize more than one free radical, they serve as the body's most potent defense against free radicals and the ensuing inflammatory reactions.

However, these antioxidants are expensive for the body to make, in terms of nutrient and energy usage. They require several different essential nutrients which can be missing from a regular American diet.

Innate antioxidants include glutathione peroxidase, catalase, coenzyme Q10, superoxide dismutase (SOD), and several more. Let's look at two of the more well-known enzyme antioxidants.

Superoxide Dismutase (SOD)

Present both inside and outside cell membranes, SOD is often called the body's "master antioxidant." It is one of the body's primary enzyme antioxidant defenses. It plays a critical role in reducing cellular oxidative stress, which is implicated in dozens of degenerative diseases.

Danish researchers have discovered that SOD binds directly to collagen, which it protects from oxidation (free radical damage). This means your entire skin and support system for joint health and mobility can be affected if you are unable to produce enough of this important antioxidant because of missing nutrient building blocks.

Some plants produce SOD. However, SOD can be destroyed by stomach acids and intestinal enzymes. Most SOD supplements are purely synthetic and nearly unassimilable. Fortunately, it is possible to boost levels of SOD through foods and supplements that supply concentrated amounts of the appropriate precursor molecules. In particular, minerals and amino acid peptides are important dietary building blocks for the body to be able to produce SOD.

Coenzyme Q10

This special enzyme antioxidant is specifically used by the mitochondria of each cell. *Mitochondria* are the energy factories of your cells, using oxygen to create the energy that fuels life. ROS free radicals are continually being produced in the mitochondria of each cell as a by-product of the energy-production process.

Mitochondrial DNA is unique to them, actually different from the DNA in your cell nucleus. The mitochondrial DNA is very vulnerable to free radical damage because of the steady stream of free radicals created by the energy production process. In order to combat them, coenzyme Q10 is produced by our body from food we eat.

CoQ10 needs to be on hand, in the mitochondria of every single cell, at all times, to neutralize these free radicals as they are formed. Its presence prevents deadly free radical damage to the mitochondrial DNA, which can potentially lead to DNA mutations and cancer.

Nutrient Antioxidants

These are antioxidants found in foods. There are two types of antioxidant foods.

Pro-antioxidant Foods

These foods contain the essential nutrient building blocks required for the production of enzyme antioxidants produced by a healthy body. These building blocks include amino acids, peptides, and trace minerals, such as copper, manganese, selenium, and zinc.

Foods with high amounts of these nutrients include sea vegetables, algae, wheatgrass, sprouted grains, seeds, and nuts.

Beyond Foods

Direct Antioxidant Foods

These foods contain nutrients that are dietary antioxidants, a type of phytonutrient. These naturally occurring antioxidants are found only in plants. They include enzymes, pigments, and hormones that plants create for their own protection and survival. These compounds give plants their color, odor, taste, and often amazing healing properties for humans.

Some, like beta-carotene, are well-known. We make vitamin A from beta-carotene. Beta-carotene is the carotenoid pigment that gives carrots their orange color, but there may be as many as six hundred different carotenoids in foods. Science is discovering that many of them are far more powerful and beneficial than even the one found in carrots.

Plants high in dietary antioxidants include green tea, wheat sprouts, algae, blueberries, and other berries (especially wild ones, such as acai), cruciferous vegetables—any edible plant with color will contain dietary antioxidants.

The most common and important antioxidants in foods include vitamins A, C, and E; all pigments; and key antioxidant families, such as catechins, flavonoids, and polyphenols.

Dietary antioxidants have their primary effect while circulating in the blood outside of the cells and are an essential component of a healthy immune system.

The Immune Connection

A large part of your body's immune system lives in your blood. White blood cells, T cells, B cells, and NK (natural killer) cells are continually circulating in order to neutralize free radicals outside cells. They "sniff out" cells under attack via chemical messengers, and assess what damage is occurring inside them. They then either fix the problem or permanently remove damaged cells.

Because your entire body sends out chemical messages to alert the immune system when cellular damage is happening, your immune system can be stressed when there are a lot of "Help Me!" signals to respond to.

Think of it like this.

You are coming up to an intersection. The light turns yellow.

On your left, an ambulance is coming with the siren on.

On the right, a fire truck has its lights flashing.

Behind you, a police officer turns on his lights and his siren.

Your cell phone rings.

The baby in the backseat begins to wail.

What do you do first?

Most of us, faced with this type of sensory overload and stress, would have a very hard time choosing what to react to first. Our ability to prioritize is compromised.

Unfortunately, what often happens with your immune system is the same; the response is either too little or way too much. When the immune system is overloaded with chemical signals for help, it can become confused and doesn't always respond correctly to the signals it is receiving.

And know this: your brain uses over 20 percent of the oxygen you breathe in. This means that your brain has a huge need for antioxidant protection against oxygen free radicals. A day without antioxidant protection can equal a day with free radical damage to brain cells.

Summary

Mental, emotional, and physical stress, along with environmental toxins, all contribute to free radical formation. When we have more ROS free radicals being formed than we can either use or neutralize, they begin their destructive cascade. ROS free radicals destroy cellular membranes, enzymes, and even our DNA.

Your body harnesses your immune system to protect cells from free radical damage. When enough antioxidants are available, many cellular free radicals are neutralized at the point of first being formed. Having enough antioxidants in your cells and bloodstream helps your immune system quell free radical damage early and prevent oxidative stress (OS).

When your body is low on antioxidant protection, your immune system spends tremendous energy in assessing cellular damage, trying to repair damage, or removing damaged cells. It is common that at this point, OS begins to cause chronic inflammation in one area or another. This is because damaged cells send out calls for help that the immune system simply cannot answer because of a lack of the raw materials necessary to accomplish the work needed.

OS can lead to overactive, underactive, or confused immune responses.

Antioxidant enzymes and *dietary antioxidants* are essential in controlling intracellular free radicals. If we have a good diet and have great health, our bodies are able to produce these powerful innate antioxidants.

Because free radicals are formed from the process of metabolism, you must be able to neutralize them quickly and efficiently throughout your body every moment of every day.

What You Can Do

Because of pollution, toxins, and stress, we have a greater need today than ever before for antioxidant nutrition.

1. Eat at least five servings of fresh fruits and colored vegetables daily.

The old adage, "An apple a day keeps the doctor away" was right! Daily consumption of a variety of fresh fruits and vegetables provides you with many beneficial antioxidants. Just add in blueberries, raspberries, tomatoes, carrots—anything with natural color.

2. Use a mineral-based sunscreen.

In my opinion, mineral sunscreens are safer than filter sunscreens, which are chemicals with irritating properties that can cause skin reactions and free radical production, especially in children.

3. Find time to play!

Stress is a huge source of free radicals. We all need time to relax and enjoy life ... and not in front of the TV!

4. Find and use a whole-food-based antioxidant supplement daily.

Not all supplements are created equal. Most people take single, isolated, and synthetic antioxidants, such as vitamins C, E, or A.

The trick to effective antioxidant supplements is to do the following:

- Use only natural whole-food complexes, enzymes, and extracts.
- Take advantage of the synergistic effect by using a whole-food formula that contains a variety of antioxidants.

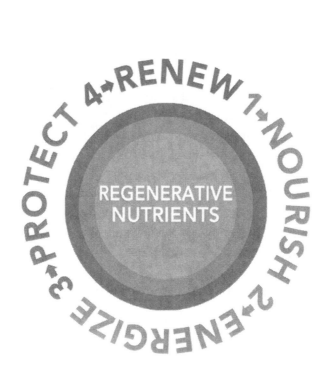

Chapter 8
Building Block 4: Regenerative Nutrients

It may be a surprise to learn you have any control at all over your genetics. It used to be that your genetics were viewed as a roll of the dice, immutable and written in your very flesh. There is some truth to this idea, but we accept that to varying degrees, genetics can be offset by lifestyle choices (i.e., altering our environment).

With environmental changes, you can minimize many genetic weaknesses, such as heart disease or diabetes. Just because your grandfather died of a heart attack at fifty-five doesn't mean you also will. You don't have to develop diabetes just because your mother is diabetic.

Beyond Foods

A common stance concerning foods and genetic tendencies is that foods are the culprits that lead to a disease. People receive the following advice.

- High-fat diets cause heart disease, so eat a low-fat diet if it runs in your family.
- Too much sugar causes diabetes, so use artificial sweeteners if diabetes runs in your family.

While there is little doubt that eating poorly will lead to health problems, especially if they run in the family (as both heart disease and diabetes often do), there is more to the food and genetics story.

Recent studies show that foods play a powerful role in how our genes are expressed. In other words, a genetic propensity for a disease or illness or a genetic strength, for that matter, *can literally be turned on or off, depending on the foods you eat.*

This goes vastly further than minimizing sugar or fats. We are talking about the potential to alter your genetic expression via the foods you eat. Eating certain foods can literally turn on the genetic link to some diseases. Eating other foods may turn those genes back off.

This field is called *nutrigenomics*.

Epigenetics

Epigenetics is the process by which the information codes stored in your chromosomes are activated or expressed. Two genetically identical people can have totally different physical experiences based on which genes are being activated or not.

Epigenetic pathways can be affected by external or internal environmental factors. Because these pathways can literally change gene expression, epigenetics is now considered an important mechanism in the cause of many diseases. It has been discovered the foods you eat—or lack—can change your epigenetics and thus, the genes that are being activated in your body.

For example, there is proof that many synthetic flavorings and ingredients adversely affect these pathways, even down the second generation. Many of the tens of thousands of flavorings developed have not been tested for long-term effects. Nutrients we extract from food also enter metabolic pathways where they are manipulated, modified, and molded into molecules the body can use.

Promoters

While most people understand DNA as being about our chromosomes, there are other parts of DNA that aren't genes and don't code for genes. Those parts are called *promoters*. Promoters are an essential epigenetic tool.

Promoters either promote or repress the decoding of a nearby gene. There are several ways promoters work to change, control, or regulate your chromosomes. One such pathway makes tags, called methyl groups, which then silence certain genes.

Silencing genes is an essential function of health. You cannot live if you constantly have every gene in every cell being activated in the same way. All the cells of your body contain *all the same* genetic codes; promoters help educate your cells as to their specific job (e.g., to be a muscle cell, a pancreatic cell, an eye cell, and so on).

Beyond Foods

The methylcobalamin form of vitamin B_{12} is absolutely essential for your chromosomes to be correctly turned on or off via promoters reading your genetic code.

A lack of B_{12} nearly guarantees you will suffer from poorly functioning genes.

Extensive studies have shown that these genetic changes can affect future generations. Children can and will inherit poor genetics from a mother's lack of B_{12}. This means the pathways your body uses to manipulate your genetic expression can be potentially handicapped your entire life because of nutrient deficiencies your mother had or you experienced in early childhood.

We can be thankful that, as adults, while a methyl-deficient (i.e., B_{12}-deficient) diet still leads to a decrease in DNA methylation, the changes are reversible when you add absorbable B_{12} back into your diet.

I want to clearly state this powerful information: what you eat, or what you lack, can turn on or off your promoters. A lack of or poorly functioning promoters can incorrectly activate or silence certain key genetic sequences. These can be genetic sequences that cause disease as well as those that could potentially prevent genetic diseases.

Telomeres

Telomeres exist at each end of a DNA strand. They are disposable sections that have no DNA or direct effect on the chromosomes they are next to. Their job is to protect the chromosomal information at the ends of the DNA strand from deteriorating or fusing with neighboring chromosomes.

Each time a cell divides to create a new replacement cell, the DNA strand is shortened as a natural part of that process. Therefore, telomeres are naturally consumed, a bit during each cell division, becoming shorter each time. If you were to completely lose the telomeres at each end of your genetic strand, the genes would progressively lose information. This could lead to cancers and other cellular malfunctions.

Therefore, when telomeres become too short, a healthy cell detects this and either stops renewing by entering a process of cellular old age (senescence) or actually begins a programmed cellular self-destruction (apoptosis).

The bottom line is as long as you have enough telomere length, your cells can continue to replicate themselves safely. This can lead to a slower aging process overall.

As we age, telomeres shorten because of many factors, many of which we have no control over. For example, there appears to be genetic coding that induces shortened telomeres as we enter the last few decades of our lives.

However, science is discovering that we *do* have control over many factors that induce telomere shortening, including:

- diet
- lifestyle choices, such as smoking
- lack of exercise
- oxidative stress

The most important of the factors we have some control over is oxidative stress. Studies indicate that telomere shortening due to free radicals has a greater absolute impact on telomere length than shortening caused by cellular aging.

Telomerase is an enzyme your body produces that increases the length of telomeres. The more telomerase your body has, the longer your cells can safely replicate. This results in cells that retain their DNA integrity for a longer time. Cells with DNA integrity result in tissues that age more slowly. Tissues that age more slowly can lead to a healthier longevity.

Scientific studies confirm that foods can directly and indirectly increase production of telomerase. In this way, your diet can add directly to your genetic health and healthy longevity.

Nucleic Acids and DNA Health

Nucleotides are the amino acid building blocks of our DNA and RNA and are found in a few foods.

RNA is the precursor to DNA and is involved in the creation of new DNA when cells divide. A lack of RNA can lead to cell death, premature aging, and cancers.

While your cells don't have to make DNA very often, they make and degrade RNA nearly continuously. RNA serves as a working copy of the genetic information sequestered in the cell nucleus and also acts as the machinery that interprets that information and uses it to produce proteins.

While you can break down the DNA and RNA in the foods you eat, your ability to absorb the nucleotides in those two nucleic acids is minimal. However, a few studies show that eating foods rich in nucleic acids (RNA and DNA) can be beneficial. Edible microalgae are one of the few foods to offer potentially usable RNA nucleotides.

It is essential is to have a diet rich in the components of nucleic acids—essential amino acids and minerals.

Adult Stem Cells

Only in the last decade has science begun to understand the key role adult stem cells play in the body's natural healthy renewal process.

What many people don't realize is there are two classifications of stem cells: those derived from embryos, called *embryonic stem cells*, and those that continue to form in our body once we are born. Called *adult stem cells*, they are produced throughout life, in large numbers when we are children and in much smaller numbers as we age.

Both embryonic and adult stem cells are capable of dividing and renewing themselves for long periods. They all have the ability to develop into any and all cell types.

Stem cells are the blank checks of your body's renewal account. They are able to become any cell your body requires—a blood cell, a skin cell, a muscle cell, or even a heart cell or brain cell.

As cells age, the DNA material inevitably becomes more fragile. At a certain point, the cell can no longer safely continue to replicate itself. At that point, a chemical signal is sent out, calling for a stem cell to replace the now dangerously old cell. Thus are we able to continue to maintain healthy cells and tissues.

During natural aging, adult stem cells have less restorative capacity and are more vulnerable to oxidative stress. This reduces the ability of the body to heal itself.

Because stem cells are the basis of ongoing renewal, their use for natural healing is profound. What is most exciting to me is that recent studies prove that foods have the ability to naturally support the body's production of healthy and vital adult stem cells. This means that with targeted formulas, you can dramatically improve the health and numbers of your own stem cells.

The fact that certain nutrients can offer great benefits and maybe even offset specific genetic diseases opens a world of possibility for being able to assume some control over your future health.

Testimonial #4: Natalie's Story

Natalie was born with Down syndrome (DS), a genetic disorder that is fairly common and therefore, well understood by the medical profession. After Natalie's birth, her mother, Lorraine, began to use whole-food supplements based on the four building blocks of functional nutrition, so that Natalie could be supplemented with great nutrients via breast milk.

At her two-month checkup, Natalie was diagnosed with a fairly severe heart defect that is common with DS. She had a large hole in her heart, and surgery was planned for as soon as she could tolerate it, since it was too large to close on its own.

Lorraine added a whole-food formula of the nutrients known to promote the health of DNA and production of adult stem cells. At three months, Natalie amazed her doctors with her development, which was on target. This is an achievement, since most infants with congenital heart defects don't thrive because of a lack of oxygen.

At four months, the cardiologist discovered the hole in her heart was healing—something he said wouldn't be possible. They delayed her surgery.

At six months, surgery was once again delayed.

At eight months, yet another large hole was found in her heart—which showed evidence of beginning to heal on its own. Natalie's heart function was clinically stronger, and her cardiologist said he had never seen a hole in this position or of this size heal on its own. He was surprised how well she was thriving, given the severity of her heart disease.

By the time Natalie was two years old, the first hole had completely healed and the second one was continuing to heal. She was small, as are most DS babies with congenital heart disease, but she was healthy and active. She was officially off any surgery list!

Natalie's story really illustrates the power of nutrients to dramatically enhance whatever strengths our genes give us.

Summary

Your genetic expression is affected through the process of *epigenetics*. Your environment, lifestyle, and dietary choices interact with your genes and can literally help you have the strongest genetics possible.

Telomerase is a natural enzyme that promotes repair of the ends of chromosomes, called telomeres, which helps your cell stay healthy and reproduce normally. Shortened telomeres signal epigenetic changes that can lead to aging.

Beyond Foods

Telomerase is active in stem cells, germ cells, hair follicles, and 90 percent of cancer cells but is low or absent in many other cells.

Cells with sufficient telomerase activity are considered immortal.

Most important to us: foods that increase telomere length in healthy cells also appear to inhibit telomerase production in cancer cells.

Adult stem cells are the true cornerstone of your body's healthy repair and rejuvenation process. Adult stem cells are found in all tissues but are especially active in bone marrow, the spleen, and a few other organs. With the right nutrients and depending on your age, your body will produce adult stem cells to replace older or dying cells, keeping your body in a state of vital health.

- Vitamin B_{12} is absolutely essential for the health of your chromosomes.
- Some foods help the longevity of your DNA.
- Foods can contain the building blocks of DNA and RNA repair.
- Foods have been proven to support your ability to produce healthy adult stem cells.

What You Can Do

Now that science is proving the powerful effects that diet and lifestyle have on our genetic code, we know we have the power to directly support healthy longevity. Lifestyle choices significantly increase telomerase activity and can also directly affect your genetic expression (epigenetic) pathways.

Lifestyle factors proven to negatively affect your DNA include:

- smoking
- excess alcohol (more than two drinks a day)
- being sedentary
- oxidative stress—this actually has a more negative effect on your DNA than any other single factor

Lifestyle factors proven to positively benefit your DNA include:

- exercise
- adequate sleep
- happiness

Foods shown to negatively affect your DNA include:

- processed meats
- baked or processed carbohydrates
- hydrogenated or trans fats
- foods cooked in high, dry heat

Foods and habits shown to benefit DNA health include:

- nutrient-dense foods that are low in calories (i.e., superfoods)
- calorie restriction, which has been shown to enhance healthy longevity
- fiber-rich foods
- antioxidant-rich foods
- vitamin-rich whole foods with essential phytonutrient vitamin cofactors
- omega-3 fatty acids found in foods, such as cold-water fish, nuts, and seeds

Beyond Foods

Foods and nutrients scientifically shown to increase the health, vitality, and production of adult stem cells include:

- blueberries
- vitamin D_3
- carnosine
- green tea / green tea extract
- omega-3 fatty acids
- AFA microalgae
- brown macroalgae

There is strong science proving that targeted formulas, in specific combinations of several of these nutrients can offer powerful, additional increases in the health and numbers of vital adult stem cells.

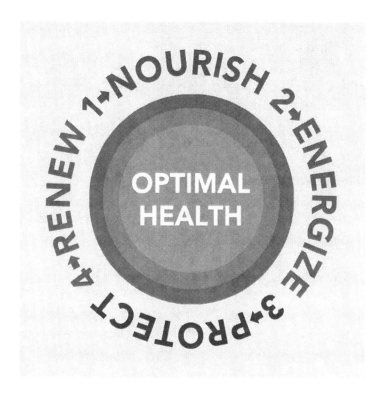

CONCLUSION

The four building blocks of functional nutrition natural healing model helps you understand some of the root causes of health issues.

Sometimes, the causes are temporary; we have a headache from working in poor light or muscle aches because we worked out too long. Other times and with all chronic problems, there is usually an underlying deficiency, imbalance, or toxicity involved.

The four building blocks help you know what foods are essential for good health. With this education and information, you are empowered to make the best food and supplement choices for your desired outcome. Use this book as a primer for ideas on simple upgrades in your diet and supplement choices, which can translate into a healthier life filled with vibrant energy.

As a last note for your empowerment, enjoy the following health facts and consider the health tips.

Here is to your long, vital, and joyous life!

Empowering Health Facts

Let's take a look at some truths that put the power of wellness back in our own hands and choices.

1. **Health is not only an absence of disease.**

Rather, disease is an end result of the absence of health and health-supporting choices. You must build health; you cannot only eliminate disease symptoms and automatically have good health.

2. **The medical model generally is a disease-focused approach.**

We cannot expect the medical process to create good health. There are actions we must take for ourselves.

3. **Many diseases are the natural result of our lifestyle and dietary choices.**

However unconscious these choices have been, we have much more power than we think to attain vitality and vibrant health.

4. **The functional nutrition approach to health views the body as a holistic system of interactive and interdependent parts.**

The digestive tract is seen as foundational to health because it is the interface between the environment and the body.

5. **The average American diet includes too many macronutrients and too few micronutrients.**

Most of us eat way too many processed foods and calories and not nearly enough whole, natural, nutrient-rich foods.

6. **Whole foods make whole people.**

Micronutrients that are found in nature (i.e., in food, especially wild or organic foods) offer us more health benefits than anything created in a chemistry lab.

7. **Eating appropriately is based on several variables, including:**
    a. condition
    b. constitution
    c. climate
    d. season
    e. age
    f. sex
    g. activity level

8. **No food is all good or bad.**

These values are relative and based on the factors listed in number 7.

9. **Every food or drink we eat or drink is either positive or negative.**

Nothing is just neutral; what we put into the body has either a negative or positive impact. The real question is how much impact it has. *No one thing we do is likely to create or destroy health.* The issue is how much or how often we do it and how many other things we are also doing that are positive or negative.

10. **Eliminating waste is as important as taking in nutrients.**

Keeping a clean digestive tract requires adequate enzymes and probiotic colonies.

Empowering Nutrition Tips

1. **What you eat occasionally isn't a problem.** What matters is what you eat daily.

2. **Listen to your inner voice.** You are the expert on your body, regardless of anyone's title or letters after his or her name.

3. **If you can't hear your inner voice or don't trust it, use the best common sense you have.** Pay attention to and learn from your own mistakes.

4. **Take guidance from others, but make your own decisions.** Take responsibility for them.

5. **Don't focus on health problems.** Focus on supporting your body's natural healing process.

6. **The natural tendency is toward health, not disease.**

7. **Include organic, wild power foods and superfoods in your diet.** This helps balance the high levels of toxicity we encounter in today's world and fills in the gaps in a nutritionally incomplete diet.

8. **A wide range of nutrients create better balance and health than having an overabundance of fewer nutrients.** Look for foods rich in multiple minerals rather than a food high in calcium alone, for example, if you want strong bones.

9. **We are not nurtured by deprivation.** The experience of eating and drinking is meant to be a nurturing human experience. Choose foods you are excited about and focus on enjoyment of what you choose.

10. **Expand your experience beyond the act of eating and drinking to include the result.** Remember that to be healthy, how you feel after consuming the food must also be enjoyable!

BIBLIOGRAPHY

The following is a partial bibliography of the books, background science, and scientific studies that support the premises of the four building blocks of functional nutrition.

1. Dr. Jeffrey Bruno, *Eat Light and Feel Bright* (2014).
2. Dr. M. Ted Morter Jr., *Your Health, Your Choice* (reprint 2012).
3. Dr. Jeffrey S. Bland, *Clinical Nutrition: A Functional Approach* (2004).
4. Steve Gagne, *Food Energetics* (2006).
5. Cooper, Dr. Kenneth H., *Advanced Nutritional Therapies* (1996).
6. The Faculty of the Harvard Medical School, Duke University Medical Center, Intellihealth.com (January 2003).
7. Allan Nation, "How We Farmed: Traditional American Farming Techniques and What We Can Learn from Them" (2005), www.westonaprice.org.
8. Ralph Martin, PhD, *Intercropping to Reduce European Corn Borer Damage*, REAP Canada (1988).
9. William A. Albrecht, PhD, *The Journal of the American Academy of Applied Nutrition* (1947).
10. L. J. Johnson, *Introductory Soil Science: A Study Guide and Laboratory Manual* (1979).
11. Barry Commoner, "How Many Harvests Do We Have Left?," Center for the Study of Biology Systems at Washington University in St. Louis, *Mother Earth News* 4 (1970).
12. Food and Agriculture Organization of the United Nations, "Conservation Agriculture: Matching Production with Sustainability," www.fao.org.
13. Joel Simmons, County Extension Agent, *Turf Net Monthly* (February 1998).
14. Stephen J. McGeady, "Immunocompetence and Allergy," *Pediatrics Magazine* (2004).

15. Jack Doyle, *Altered Harvest* (1985).
16. Cambridge Experimentation Review Board (January 1977).
17. S. Wright, *Molecular Politics Developing American and British Regulatory Policy for Genetic Engineering, 1972–1982* (Chicago: University of Chicago Press, 1996).
18. E. Ann Clark, "Environmental Risks of GE: Why You Should Take Them Seriously," Presented to the Forum of the Toronto Biotechnology Initiative, April 15, 1999, Toronto, ON.
19. Janet F. Davidson, and Michael S. Sweeney, *On the Move: Transportation and the American Story* (2003).
20. Eric Schlosser, *Fast Food Nation: The Dark Side of the All-American Meal* (2001).
21. Dr. Elias Metchnikoff, *Prolongation of Life* (1916).
22. Robert Parson, "Ozone Depletion FAQ Part IV: UV Radiation and Its Effects" (1997), www.faqs.org.
23. I. N. Acworth, and B. Bailey, *The Handbook of Oxidative Metabolism*, Massachusetts: ESA Inc. (1997).
24. John Papaconstantineau, PhD, Sealy Center for Molecular Science (2004), www.scms.utmb.edu/faculty/papa/.
25. Mayo Clinic Health Letter, "Whole foods: What They Give You That Supplements Can't" (August 1998).
26. Jordan Rubin, *The Townsend Letter for Doctors and Patients* (February—March 2004).
27. Food & Nutrition Board, National Academy of Sciences, National Research Council, Washington DC, Men (M) and Women (W), 1989 28, *Metabolism* 50 no. 7 (July 2001): 767–70.
28. Gary Price Todd, MD, *Nutrition, Health & Disease* (1985).
29. Stephen E. Whiting, PhD, *Not All Minerals Are Created Equal*, HealingWithNutrition.com (1999).
30. DeWayne Ashmead, *Chelated Mineral Nutrition in Plants, Animals, and Man* (1982).
31. Senate Document 264, 1936.

32. Janet Hunt, PhD, RD, and Johanna Dwyer, DSc, RD, "Food Fortification and Dietary Supplements," *Journal of the American Dietetic Association* (2001).
33. Heather L. Van Epps, "Eating Oily Fish May Reduce Inflammation," *Journal of Experimental Medicine* (March 2005).
34. L. G. Cleland, M. J. James, H. Keen, D. Danda, G. Caughey, and S. M. Proudman, "Fish Oil—An Example of an Anti-Inflammatory Food," *Asia Pacific Journal of Clinical Nutrition* (2005).
35. J. A. Vinson, "Comparative Bioavailability of Synthetic and Natural Vitamin C in Guinea Pigs," *Nutrition Reports International* 27, no. 4 (1983): 875–880.
36. G. W. Burton, M. G. Traber, R.V. Acuff, et al., "Human Plasma and Tissue ATocopherol Concentrations in Response to Supplementation with Deuterated Natural and Synthetic Vitamin E," *American Journal of Clinical Nutrition* (1998) 67: 669–684.
37. Ron Kennedy, MD, *A Short History of Vitamins*, The Doctor's Medical Library (2005).
38. Patrick Rump, Ronald P. Mensink, Arnold D. M. Kester, and Gerard Hornstra, "Essential Fatty Acid Composition of Plasma Phospholipids and Birth Weight: A Study in Term Neonates," *American Journal of Clinical Nutrition* (April 2001).
39. D. F. Horrobin, "Essential Fatty Acids in Clinical Dermatology," *Journal of the American Academy of Dermatology* (June 1989).
40. M. Haag, "Essential Fatty Acids and the Brain," *Canadian Journal of Psychiatry* (April 2003).
41. Carmia Borek, PhD, "Fish and the N-3 Fatty Acids Reduce Risk of Alzheimer's Disease," *Life Extension Magazine* (November 2003).
42. Jane Higdon, *Discover Magazine* (February 2003).
43. A. J. Gelenberg, "Tyrosine for the Treatment of Depression," *American Journal of Psychiatry* (May 1980).
44. A. Singhal, MD, K. Kennedy, MSc, J. A. Lanigan, BSc, and A. Lucas, MD, "Effect of Dietary Nucleotides on the Intestinal

Flora of Healthy Term Infants," *Journal of Parenteral and Enteral Nutrition* (January–February 2004).
45. The Faculty of the Harvard Medical School, Intellihealth.com.
46. Y. Ishida, F. Nakamura, H. Kanzato, D. Sawada, H. Hirata, A. Nishimura, O. Kajimoto, and S. Fujiwara, "Clinical Effects of *Lactobacillus acidophilus* Strain L-92 on Perennial Allergic Rhinitis: A Double-Blind, Placebo-Controlled Study," The American Dairy Science Association (2005).
47. "GERD in America," Louis Harris and Associates survey (1997).
48. P. Wahlqvist, "Symptoms of Gastroesophageal Reflux Disease, Perceived Productivity & Health-Related Quality of Life," *American Journal of Gastroenterology* (August 2001).
49. M. A. Eloubeidi, and D. Provenzale, "Health-Related Quality of Life and Severity of Symptoms in Patients with Barrett's Esophagus and Gastroesophageal Reflux Disease Patients without Barrett's Esophagus," *American Journal of Gastroenterology* (August 2000).
50. Joseph Pizzorno, ND, *Total Wellness: Improve Your Health by Understanding the Body's Healing Systems* (1996).
51. Dixie Farley, *Taming Tummy Turmoil*, FDA *Consumer* (June 1995).
52. Sidney Wolfe, MD, *Best Pills, Worst Pills* (2009).
53. National Museum of Science and Industry, "Enzymes," www.sciencemuseum.org.uk (2005).
54. *Encyclopedia Britannica*, "Enzymes" (2003).
55. Nicole M. de Roos, and Martijn B. Katan, *Effects of Probiotic Bacteria on Diarrhea, Lipid Metabolism, and Carcinogenesis: A Review of Papers Published between 1988 and 2006.*
56. Kevin J. Barnham, Colin L. Masters, and Ashley I. Bush, "Neurodegenerative Diseases and Oxidative Stress," *Nature Reviews Drug Discovery* 3 (2004): 205–214.
57. T. Finkel, and N. J. Holbrook, "Oxidants, Oxidative Stress and the Biology of Aging," *Nature* 408 (2000): 239, 247.

58. Barry Halliwell, and John M.C. Gutteridge, *Free Radicals in Biology and Medicine*, Oxford Science Publications (1999).
59. D. Pratico, "Alzheimer's Disease and Oxygen Radicals: New Insights," *Biochemical Pharmacology* (February 2002).
60. P. C. Calder, and S. Kew, "The Immune System: A Target for Functional Foods?," *The British Journal of Nutrition* (2002).
61. Joy E. Swanson, PhD, "What Are Antioxidants?," Cornell Cooperative Extension, Division of Nutritional Sciences, Cornell University (1999).
62. Mike Adams, "Canadian Cancer Society Announces National Program to Prevent Cancer Using Vitamin D," June 11, 2007, http://www.newstarget.comVitamin_D.html.
63. Joan Lappe, PhD, RN, "Creighton Study Shows Vitamin D Reduces Cancer Risk," June 8, 2007, http://www2.creighton.edu/publicrelations/newscenter/news/2007/june2007/june82007/vitamind_cancer_nr060807/index.php.
64. Sunlightnews.com.
65. Maureen Ryan, "Screen Test: Reading the Micro-Fine Print," *The Green Guide*, May 22, 2007.
66. Virginia Culler, *Chemical Sunscreens—When Are We Safe?*, http://serendip.brynmawr.edu/biology/b103/f02/web1/vculler.html.
67. USDA, Agricultural Statistics 2005.
68. "Monsanto Versus Percy Schmeiser," www.grist.org/advice/ask/2006/05/24/canola/.
69. Ghafoor Unisa, "Fats in Indian Diets and Their Nutritional and Health Implications," *Lipids* (1996): 5287–5291.
70. I. Shenolikar, "Fatty Acid Profile of Myocardial Lipid in Populations Consuming Different Dietary Fats," *Lipids* (1980): 980–982.
71. J. F. Bellenand, G. Baloutch, N. Ong, and J. Lecerf, "Effects of Coconut Oil on Heart Lipids and on Fatty Acid Utilization in Rapeseed Oil," *Lipids* (1980): 938–943.

72. M. Indu, and M. Ghafoor Unisa, "N-3 Fatty Acids in Indian Diets—Comparison of the Effects of Precursor (Alpha-Linolenic Acid) Vs. Product (Long Chain N-3 Poly Unsaturated Fatty Acids)," *Nutrition Research* (1992): 569–582.
73. B. Gesch, S. Hammond, S. Hampson, et al., "Influence of Supplementary Vitamins, Minerals and Essential Fatty Acids on the Antisocial Behaviour of Young Adult Prisoners," *British Journal of Psychiatry* 181 (July 2002): 22–8.
74. Dr. Lukas Rist, *British Journal of Nutrition*.
75. Jay Olshansky, PhD, Douglas J. Passaro, MD, Ronald C. Hershaw, MD, Jennifer Layden, MPH, Bruce A. Carnes, PhD, Jacob Brody, MD, Leonard Hayflick, PhD, Robert N. Butler, MD, David B. Allison, PhD, and David S. Ludwig, MD, PhD, "A Potential Decline in Life Expectancy in the United States in the 21st Century," *The New England Journal of Medicine* (March 17, 2005).
76. *Psychiatric Services*, A Journal of the American Psychiatric Association (April 2004).
77. Department of Health and Human Services.
78. American Academy of Child and Adolescent Psychiatry.
79. *British Medical Journal* (2006).
80. Deborah Lott, "Childhood Trauma, CRF Hypersecretion and Depression," *Psychiatric Times* 16 (October 1999): 10.
81. "Myths of Depression Challenged," *Psychiatric Times* (2000).
82. A. Robert Parson, "Ozone Depletion FAQ Part IV: UV Radiation and its Effects" (1997).
83. I. N. Acworth, and B. Bailey, *The Handbook of Oxidative Metabolism* (Massachusetts: ESA Inc., 1997).
84. National Academies of Sciences, *US Health in International Perspective: Shorter Lives, Poorer Health* (2013).
85. Claire M. Hasler, PhD, *Functional Foods: Their Role in Disease Prevention and Health Promotion*, Institute of Food Technologies.

86. Dairy Council of California, *The Quest for Optimal Health: What You Need to Know about Functional Foods.*
87. Richardson Centre for Functional Foods and Nutraceuticals, "Vision and Mandate," (2009).
88. Agriculture and Agri-Food Canada, *What Are Functional Foods and Nutraceuticals?* (April 2009).
89. Alan E. Nourse, and the Editors of *LIFE*, *The Body*, Life Science Library (1961).
90. Chemistry GCSe Passbook, "Key Facts" (1988).
91. Walter Mertz, MD, *Implications of the New Trace Elements for Human Health*, US Department of Agriculture, SEA, HN, Nutrition Institute.
92. Karl H. Schutte, PhD, and John A. Myers, MD, *Metabolic Aspects of Health*, Nutritional Elements in Health and Disease (1979).
93. Steven H. Harvey, *Minerals: Right on Target, Studies in the Use of Pure Amino Acid Chelated Mineral Supplements, Based on the Research of Dr. Harvey Ashmead*, Nature's Field (1987).
94. Soir A. Smolin, and Mary B. Grosvenor, *Nutrition Science & Applications* (1994).
95. Jeffrey Bland, PhD, "The Trace Mineral Revolution in Human Health," *The Digest of Chiropractic Economics* (May/June 1980).
96. Dr. Wayne Ashmead, PhD, "Without Chelation—You're Dead," *World Health & Ecology* (1976).
97. *Science Daily*, "Studies on Nutrients, Gene Expression Could Lead to Tailored Diets for Disease Prevention," http://www.sciencedaily.com/releases/2010/03/100305112159.htm.
98. *Science Daily*, "New Study Links DHA Type of Omega-3 to Better NervousSystem Function," http://www.sciencedaily.com/releases/2009/12/091216130718.htm.
99. Beth Saltman, "Nature's Barcode Tells the Story of Foods' True Origin," http://www.npr.org/blogs/thesalt/2012/04/03

/149921493/natures-barcodetells-the-story-of-foods-true-origin?sc=tw.
100. D. Ghadimi, R. Foister-Holst, M. de Vrese, P. Winkler, K. J. Heller, and J. Schrezenmeir, "Effects of Probiotic Bacteria and Their Genomic DNA on TH 1/TH2-Cytokine Production by Peripheral Blood Mononuclear Cells (Pbmcs) of Healthy and Allergic Subjects," *Immunobiology* (2008).
101. Y. Zhong, J. Huang, W. Tang, B. Chen, and W. Cai, "Effects of Probiotics, Probiotic DNA and the CPG Oligodeoxynucleotides on Ovalbumin-Sensitized Brown-Norway Rats Via TLR9/NF-B Pathway," *FEMS Immunol Med Microbiology* 66 no. 1 (October 2012):71–82.

CPSIA information can be obtained at www.ICGtesting.com
Printed in the USA
LVOW08s1212300516

490437LV00004B/419/P